Withanage Series In Surgery

Wound Care and Management

DR ATHULA WITHANAGE

MD PYDH. LMSSA London.

FRCS Edinburgh. FRCS Ireland. FRCS England. FICS

Retired Lead Clinician Department of Surgery WGH. Hywel Dda NHS University Trust.

Piyaseeli Withanage Charity Trust Surgeon. Asian Sector & Consultant Wound Care Specialist (WGH & CETH)

Consultant General & Laparoscopic Surgeon.

Senior Lecturer in Surgery. Hon. Clinical Tutor Cardiff University.

Faculty WIMAT, Cardiff , University of Wales.

SAITM & KDU. Clinical Supervisor, Educational Supervisor & Examiner.

Colombo East Teaching Hospital

Preface

The aim of this book is to give an insight about modern concepts of wound care and an up to date account of wound management. Every medical student, junior doctor, nurse practitioner, wound care specialist at various level of medical education need to know the fundamentals of wound care. I believe that This will be a very useful book to be kept in all wound care departments. I have provided essential information, without over burdening the medical student and all wound care practitioners. Hopefully based on the information in this book, healthcare facilities countrywide can have a unified and consistent approach to wound care and conduct and disseminate local research, for all healthcare practitioners to follow.

It is of paramount importance that we do not cause harm to the healing wound and to the peri-wound skin by our treatment. It is also vital that we have a holistic approach to wound management by paying attention to the patient's overall condition and his or her social background.

I hope we can update this book from time to time with the help of my colleagues in the field to keep up with modern research and developments. The readers are requested to send suggestions for improvement of the book which will be incorporated in future prints. Please communicate any comments, shortcomings etc. to me at athulawithanage@hotmail.co.uk

I would like to thank Dr. Nelun de Silva, Consultant Microbiologist at Colombo East Teaching Hospital for editing the book. I am grateful to Dr. Chaminda Kumara and Dr. Sahani Croos for collecting data and photographs from our practice at CETH. Finally I like to thank my wife Nelum for typing the book.

Athula Withanage MD.FRCS.

"Embrace hope – wounds are curable"

Dedicated to

Peoples Friendship University. Russia.

On the occasion of 60th anniversary' 8 th February 2020.

My wife Nelumkanthi, and children Triona, Shanuka and Dylan.

Celebrating 50 years of Service to Public & National Health,
Medical education and 25 years of Surgical skill training for
RCS.

Three times nominee for the prestigious Silver Scalpel Award
for the best surgical trainer of the year and twicw winner of
Clinical Leader and Mentor of the year award (2008 & 2009)

CONTENT

Introduction

Healing refers to the replacement of destroyed tissue by living tissue in the body. It is the mechanism through which the body repairs and restores the integrity of damaged tissues. It is a complex interaction of physical, chemical, and cellular events and is essential for the survival of the individual and to maintain quality of life. An understanding of the healing process, especially its various stages is essential if wounds are to be properly assessed and their management is planned.

The usage of betadine alone for any stage of wound healing has been overused and misused. This causes delay in wound healing and considerable pain to the patient.

The author has seen bilateral varicose ulcers being dressed with betadine for over 2 years in a patient where the wound was regularly dressed with betadine soaked gauze. There were no signs of wound healing and the patient required narcotic analgesia. Just by substituting the dressing to hydrocolloid gel the pain subsided and afterwards varicose veins surgery was performed to deal with the etiological factor and the wound healed within 6 weeks.

The main aim of this book is to provide guidelines and to identify a unified and consistent approach to the management of wound care across the island for all practitioners to follow. It is vital to select the correct dressing for the appropriate stage of wound healing.

The old concept of encouraging drying up of wounds with scab formation has now been largely abandoned as the modern concept of wound healing is to retain appropriate moisture in the wound. This is to promote natural healing process by maintaining a warm moist and nontoxic environment. Aim is to "do no harm" or injury to wound or surrounding peri-wound tissues by using safe, simple, cost effective, non-irritant, non-allergenic dressings and treatments. In the use of wound dressings, it is important not to traumatize new tissues on removal, to minimise frequency of dressing change and to have a good rationale and evidence base for their use.

Wound Healing Matrix (WHM);

For assessment, classification and diagnosis, the term Wound Healing Matrix proposed by wound healing research unit is very useful. This has been modified to reflect the overall condition of the patient.

Modified Wound Healing Matrix (WHM) has six components;

1. Site

The site will determine what tissues or combination of tissues is involved in the wound.

Skin	–	Epidermis and dermis
Bone	–	Simple closed or open compound fractures.
		Blood vessels- arterial or venous
Nerves	–	Central and peripheral.
Bowel	–	Oesophagus, gastric, large bowel and small bowel.
Tubular structures	–	bile, lacrimal, pancreatic, salivary ducts, ureters and urethra
Solid organs	–	liver, spleen and kidney -

2. Aetiology

a. Acute wounds.

Trauma   –   Direct or indirect-

Surgery   –   Elective or emergency -

Thermal, chemical or radiation Injury

Pressure and friction; pressure sores.

Ischemia and infarct

Inflammation and abscess formation

b. Chronic wounds

Vascular ulcers; venous (stasis), arterial (ischemic) and mixed

Pressure sores; treatment varies depending on the four classes(described later) of pressure sores as well as the general management of the bedridden emaciated patient with anaemia and poor nutrition.

Diabetic Ulcer; the foot may be neuropathic (warm foot), ischemic (Cold foot) or neuro-ischaemic. Major part of management consists of control of diabetes.

Malignant ulcer; Marjolins ulcer (A chronically inflamed ulcer with gross scaring e.g. long standing venous ulcer). For malignant ulcers an incision biopsy at the edge including normal skin is essential to exclude Squamous cell carcinoma or Basal cell carcinoma (Rodent ulcer).

Infective ulcers; Tuberculosis, tropical ulcer; synergistic gangrene.

Management consist of treatment of the aetiology as well as local treatment of ulcers. In long standing ulcers exclusion of malignancy by biopsy is important.

3. Phases of wound healing.

Wound healing is a dynamic process which can be divided into three phases. It is important to remember that it is not a linear process and there is considerable overlap. Sometimes it is delayed in one of the stages or can reverse back or rapidly go through all three stages at a speed depending upon extrinsic or intrinsic factors within the patient. It is important to know in what stage the wound is in when first seen.

Haemostasis to stop bleeding (coagulation phase) is the beginning of the healing process following any injury or surgical incision.

I. Inflammatory phase post trauma. Cleaning and repair cells and growth factors move to the site.

II. Proliferative phase - Pink or red granulation tissue formation, rapid epithelialisation occurs in moist and appropriately hydrated wounds.

III. Maturation phase. This is the remodelling stage of wound healing.

These phases will be described in more detail later. (Chapter 03)

4. Clinical manifestations

A description of the ulcer or the wound should include the following:

types of tissues involved

- site
- size
- floor
- base
- presence of sinuses
- shape that may cause problems when choosing the treatment or dressings.

- dry or wet
- amount of discharge
- clean or infected,
- dry necrotic or wet gangrenous.

Assessment of the wound is of paramount importance before any treatment is recommended.

Following features also should be taken into account:
- Bleeding
- Epithelialisation
- granulation or exuberant over granulation formation (Proud Flesh)
- foul smelling or not
- presence of major vital structures such as blood vessels in the base or in the vicinity of the wound

Fistulae formation, especially the fistulas that are communicating with internal organs or peritoneal cavity are particularly important.

5. Environment and Care givers

This will affect the choice of treatment and length of time of hospitalisation. Some methods such as maggot therapy or negative pressure treatment. i.e. Vacuum Assisted Closure (VAC Therapy) may not be available in the community outside the hospital.

In the hospital environment, wound care specialist should be a Doctor, preferably with some vascular interest or a nurse specialist trained in wound care. It is vital to establish a well-equipped wound care department. Special reclining chairs with leg stands, proper lighting, shower trays, tanks with drainage systems, dressing and dissecting packs with gloves should be available.

In the community, Old People's Home or Nursing Homes; a district or community nurse or a trained carer should attend. In the patient's home, a district nurse or non-trained family carer or self-care can be provided. Carer can work for some time under the supervision of the nurse until she or he can take over the management at home.

Regular visits by GPs should be organised and if necessary requests can be made for Hospital consultant for joint domiciliary visits.

6 Patient's clinical condition

The important factors to be considered are, the patients nutrition level, age, whether the patent is disabled or not (severe rheumatoid arthritis or paralysed patient-post stroke or bed ridden due to any other condition). Other co-morbid factors such as bleeding diatheses, whether the patient is on anticoagulant or antiplatelet therapy should be looked into because during wound debridement, maggot therapy or VAC therapy, bleeding from the site may increase. The past medical history such as malignancy, renal impairment etc. are also important.

Chapter 2

Principles of wound care – Primary aims.

The primary aims should be to:

(1) Promote and support natural healing process.

(2) Create and maintain an ideal wound environment – A moist wound healing environment: concept promoted by George Winter[1].

(3) Prevent secondary damage as well as iatrogenic damage caused by materials used for dressings, injudicious, inappropriate dressing change.

(4) Irrigate the wound with appropriate warm solutions and avoid cold lavage which will delay healing.

(5) Use an ideal dressing which is non-irritant, non-allergenic and non - traumatic. It is important to get a proper history in relation to previous treatment and dressings.

(6) Evaluate, plan and implement wound care with consideration for the individual patient and not just the wound. To do this it is of paramount importance to assess aetiological factors, other co-morbidities and patient's social background.

---

1 (Winter G D formation of scab and rate of epithelisation of superficial wounds in the shin of the young domestic pig. Nature 1962; 193: 293 – 294)

(7) Give care and attention to social and psycho-sexual problems, associated with wounds on the face, neck, breast, abdomen and genitalia.

(8) Maintain privacy and confidentiality, respect patient's culture, religious beliefs and patient's choice.

Chapter 3

Normal wound healing

Healing is the mechanism through which the body repairs and restores the integrity of damaged tissues. Clear understanding of this process is essential if wounds are to be accurately assessed and correct management is introduced. There is no one method of treatment which fits every patient or the wound.

In this context it is important to know the three basic types of cells in the body.

a. Labile Cells;

These are continuously dividing cells e.g. skin epithelial cells and bone marrow cells.

b. Quiescent Cells;

These cells undergo rapid division in response to injury. E.g. parenchymal cells of liver, kidney and pancreas, mesenchymal cells of the smooth muscles, fibroblasts and vascular endothelial cells.

c. Permanent Cells;

These cells cannot undergo mitotic division in post-natal life. E.g. nerve cells, skeletal and cardiac muscle cells.

The normal healing processes go through three classical overlapping phases. This is an orchestrated series of events which takes place in the wounded area. Healing is influenced by local as well as systemic factors.

1. Inflammatory Phase: 0 – 3 days.

After injury, the initial response is haemostasis. This applies to both traumatic wounds as well as operative incisional wounds. Haemostasis begins with vasoconstriction and activation of clotting and complement cascade.

The smaller vessels in the wound thrombose, some go into spasm and bleeding stops spontaneously. In surgical incisional wounds, vasoconstriction and haemostatic platelet plug formation is the only process involved. The surgeon may also help the process by cautery or ligation of bleeding vessels in the vicinity. One must be careful not to leave tissue ligation stumps too long and large areas of cauterised tissues in the wound as they eventually become necrotic, leading to sloughing and infection.

Platelets adhere to the damaged endothelium, releasing adenosine di-phosphate which causes further thrombocytic aggregation. This interaction requires Von-Willebrand factor in the plasma. This factor is also released by endothelial cells. As a result of this process, blood vessels thromboses and bleeding stops. Extravasated blood also coagulates. True inflammatory phase then follows with cell recruitment via chemotaxis.

When bleeding stops, platelets activate and de-granulate (alpha-granules). Platelet derived growth factors [(PDGF, platelet factor four, and transforming growth factor beta (TGF beta[2])] are involved in the process.[2]

In the inflammatory reaction; Cytokines cause a major influence. (Slavin 1999). The classic description of Celsius AD in the first century described the symptoms and signs as – Rubor (redness),

2. (Holmson R Day HJ, Stormoken 1969. The blood platlelet release reaction J Haematology Suplt 8; 1 – 26).

Tumor (swelling), Calor (heat) and Dolor (pain) and Functio laesa (loss of function) was later added by Galen. Patients lying in bed with visibly red, painful, warm swelling is what we see every day in our clinical practice e.g. cellulitis of limbs, infected wounds, boils.

Coagulation consists of conversion of soluble fibrinogen into insoluble fibrin. This conversion is catalysed by thrombin (precursor – prothrombin). Conversion of factor X to Xa requires factor X11 initiated intrinsic pathway or Tissue Factor initiated extrinsic pathway.

The mechanism that produces the fibrin clot;

Exist in blood – intrinsic pathway.   Extrinsic (To blood) following tissue damage

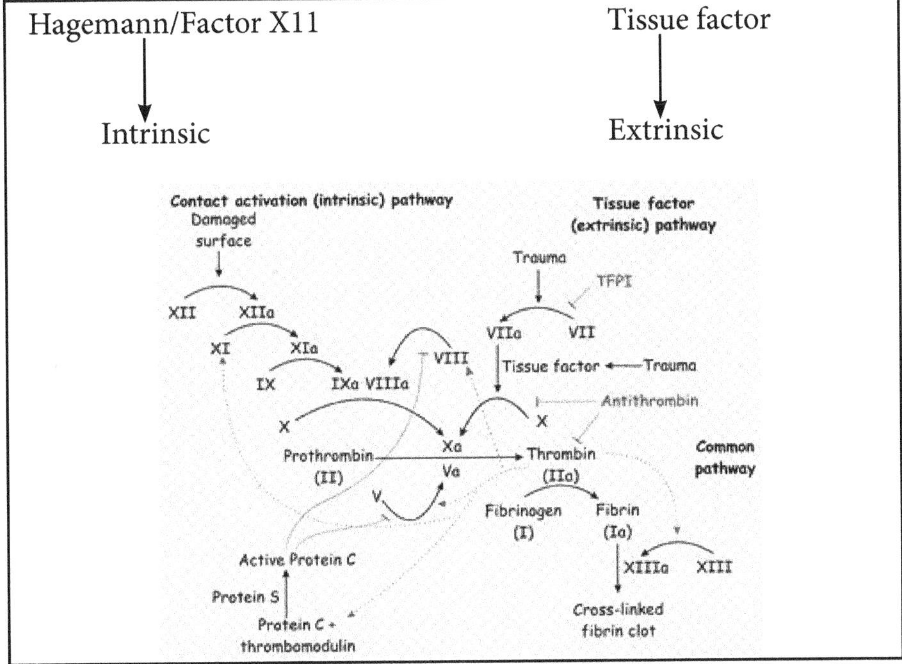

Inactive Fibrinolysis system also activate for the dissolution of clot following injury and clotting.

Complement System

Fragments of Hageman's factor and Bradykinin initiates the complement system. They are a series of inter-reacting soluble proteins found in serum and extracellular fluids[3].

Complement system forms a membrane attack complex-MAC (C5b, C6, C7, C8, C9) potentially a cytolytic complex to promote lysis of target cells i.e. pathogens. This is a potent mechanism contributing to innate defence against pathogens.

Opsonisation of bacteria with complement C3b will result in phagocytosis by macrophages.

Alternative pathway of the complement system is to amplify the local inflammatory response.

In the wound neutrophils which have a short lifespan reach a maximum in 24 to 48 hours. Their function is phagocytosis of bacteria. (The soldiers).

Macrophages (the support troops) appear 2 – 3 days after injury. Macrophages clear devitalised tissues, dead white cells, microorganisms and regulate fibroblast activity.

Growth factors that are liberated, target various cells in the wound and act on all three phases promoting matrix synthesis, angiogenesis and epithelialisation. Growth factors are now increasingly used in the wound healing.

2. Proliferative phase (3 – 21 days)

Fibroblasts recruited probably from local mesenchymal cells proliferate to reach peak on the 7th day. They synthesise extracellular proteins, growth factors and angiogenic factors.

---

3 (Chery At El 1994. Chery G Huges, Kingsworth AN; Arnold F Wound healing in Morris PJ and Maul RA 1994 edition. Oxford textbook of surgery volume 1. Oxford University Press).

This phase is characterized by formation of granulation tissue in the wound space. Looks shiny wet puffy pinkish red to the naked eye and bleed easily when touched. It is made from inflammatory cells, new capillary loops in a loose extracellular matrix (ECM).

ECM is made of adhesive proteins such as fibronectins or laminins, fibrous proteins such as collagens and elastins, and polysaccharides such as proteoglycans and glucose-aminoglycans

Collagens (80%) made by fibroblast are the most abundant proteins in animal tissues anywhere in the body.

It has four types. Types 1 and 3 contribute to the tensile strength of the wound. Collagen synthesis and degradation is finely balanced[4].

For angiogenesis, endothelial cells come from the edges of the wound. This process is influenced by angiogenic factors including fibroblast growth factor (FGF). Knob like capillaries sprout from existing small vessels at the wound edge. They meet in the centre of the wound and connect.[5]

Macrophages secretes angiogenic factors, under early hypoxic conditions of the wound. Other cytokines may also be involved in the process[6].

Invasion of new capillaries into the fibrin clot is known as invasive angiogenesis. Integrins inhibit invasive angiogenesis and granulation tissue formation.

Integrins are part of the group of adhesion molecules embedded into the cell membrane. These molecules bind cells to extra cellular matrix involved with transmembrane cell signalling (outside in or inside

4 (Slaving J 1999 wound healing and pathophysiology – Surgery 17 to 41 Volume).

5 (Ausprunk DH; Folkman J. 1997. Migration and proliferation of endothelial cells in preformed and newly formed blood vessels during tumour angiogenesis. Microvascular Research 14, 53 – 65).

6(Knighton et al 1983 – oxygen tension regulates the expression of angiogenesis factor by macrophages – Science 221; 1283 – 1285).

out). They are proteins which comprise of alpha and beta which act as receptors that mediate cell to cell and cell to matrix interactions[7].

Elastin (2 – 4 %) provides elasticity and resilience.

Fibronectin, a high molecular weight adhesion glycoprotein of the extracellular matrix that binds to membrane spanning integrins. They play a role in re-modelling as a mediator between cells and collagen.

Proteoglycans form an extremely well hydrated gel which forms the ground substance. They act as fillers between the spaces that occur between cells.

The role of Matrix Metalloproteinases

Protein degradation also takes place by proteases (metalloproteinases) secreted by the local cells in the wound. They are proteases found in combination with metal ions - Zn2+

Neutrophil derived matrix metalloproteinase 8 (MMP 8) is the predominate collagenase present in healing wounds. Over expression and activation of MMP 8 maybe involved in the pathogenesis in non-healing chronic wounds helped by the low levels of Tissue Inhibitor Metalloproteinase 1 (TIMP 1)[8].

Balance between protein synthesis and degradation will determine successful healing or fibrosis of a wound. Loss of MMP regulation is characteristic of chronic wounds and contributes to slowing down or failure to heal.

Epithelialisation

Marginal basal epithelial cell loses its cohesion from the underlying dermis and migrate in "leap – frog" fashion across the wound centripetally. Contact inhibition takes place when they meet in the centre. Then a new basement membrane is slowly regenerated[9]

7 (Slaving J 1999 wound healing and pathophysiology – surgery 17 to 41 Volume).
8(J Am Podiatr,Med. Assoc Jan; 92(1); 12-8).
9 (Moulin V (1995) growth factors in skin wound healing – Eu. J. Cell Biology 68, 1 – 7).

In sutured, steri-stripped, glued or clipped (stapled) wounds which are perfectly apposed, epithelial migration is completed within 72 hours. This is the most vulnerable time for the wound. It is important to remember change of dressing is unnecessary during this time and will be detrimental (Injudicious dressing change).

It is important to remember that epithelium only migrate over live "moist" tissues. If debris, slough, necrotic tissue or foreign body is present, epithelialisation will be delayed or may never take place. Hence creating a proper environment by wound debridement is of paramount importance. Optimum epithelialisation occurs in moist environment (G Winter 1962). It can proceed under a dry scab but at a very slower rate. This was clearly demonstrated by Winter in animal experiments. This is the modern concept of wound healing.

Wound contraction

Wound contraction starts from 5th day post injury. The force is provided by contractile ability of fibroblast and myofibroblast. This mechanism is important in wounds with appreciable tissue loss. Integrins may take part in binding collagen to produce a network which pulls the wound edges together. Linear wounds shorten and the circular wounds (Urethra, bowel, bile ducts) narrow sometimes to produce stenosis or stricture.

There are two theories –

(1) Myofribroblast Cell Contraction Theory

According to this theory myofibroblasts contracts like a muscle.

(2) Fibroblast Cell – Traction Theory.

Here the mechanism is lattice like contraction and is appears to be related to cell locomotion.

In the case of Myofibroblast, mechanism is based upon cell contractions only. This theory explains the wound contraction as a tank – thread like traction, by the cell on the Matrix[10].

3. Maturation and Re-modelling Phase(7 days to one year)

Fibronectin, hyaluronic acid and proteoglycans in ECM provides provisional fibre network. Subsequently collagen deposition, redistribution and re-orientation take place. Type I collagen replaces Type III in 4: 1 ratio.

Tensile strength of the wound increases to 50% in 6 weeks. Maximum strength gain is about 70%. Cross matching of suture strength (tensile strength) with tissue strength during healing is important in order to maintain integrity of tissues. Tensile strength is the stability of the suture which enables it to withstand the forces exerted on it during healing.

Collagen synthesis as well as degradation takes place simultaneously. Degradation is due to collagenases. Cellularity and also vascularity reduces. Dusky reddish appearance of the new scar and changes to the familiar pale whitish scar tissue.

Scar is the final outcome of wound healing and is responsible for continuity, strength and function of the tissues.

Peripheral Nerve Injury, axonal degeneration and regeneration.

Nerve cells cannot divide or regenerate but degenerated axons can regenerate distally into the surviving neurilemmal sheath or tube, if the sheath is accurately constructed. When any nerve is cut, anti-grade axonal injury takes place, and retrograde traumatic degeneration up to the next node of Ranvier (myelin sheath gap) also occurs.

10(Earlich R F Rajarathnam. JBM 1990. Cell locomotion forces vs cell contraction forces for collagen lattice contraction. An in-vitro model for wound contraction tissue and cell; 22; 407 – 417).

Macrophages and Schwann Cells actively clear the sheath. Axonal tip or sprout draws into the neurilemmal sheath if properly or perfectly guided by surgical intervention. The growth is very slow and is about one millimetre a day. Perhaps it is best not to promise the patient that all will be normal when the external wound is healed. Nerve regeneration can be assessed crudely by immersing hands in cold water for 20 minutes (just an observation made in plastic surgery clinic, Professor. O'Rian St.Vincents Hospital Dublin.). The normally sensitive areas will wrinkle as normal skin does. The area can be mapped to see the progress in follow up clinics. A painful neuroma may form at its tip if neurilemmal sheath is not properly approximated. Problem of mix up of sensory or motor fibres does exist. Schwann cells also provide the substrate for axonal regeneration. After regeneration, re-myelination takes place. This process is regulated by neurotropic and other growth factors.

Factors affecting wound healing

(1) Age – Wound healing alter with age. It is the risk factor which cannot be modified. As we get older all three classical phases become much slower. The collagen production and angiogenesis proceeds at a slower speed. Epithelialisation takes a long time to develop.

(2) Uraemia - is associated with malnutrition and general inhibition of proliferation of all types of cells involved with healing.

(3) Anaemia –Anaemia delays healing due to poor supply of oxygen. Factors which cause anaemia on their own may delay wound healing. E.g. Malignancy, poor nutritional status.

(4) Jaundice - Fibronectin contents of extracellular matrix is reduced in jaundice. High levels of bilirubin itself reduce fibroblast multiplications.

(5) Diabetes – In diabetic micro-angiopathy with thickened basement membrane and capillary steal syndrome due to proximal shunting, cause ischaemia of distal tissues. In diabetic neuropathy, insensitive skin is more liable to trauma of friction and pressure. Formation of abnormal collagen cause tissue breakdown. Hyperglycaemia also reduces the activity of leucocytes, macrophages and in turn lowers the fibroblast production. In Diabetes, wounds are more susceptible to infections. Atherosclerosis obviously goes hand in hand in diabetes and causes additional ischaemia.

(6) Steroids – As well as reducing the inflammatory response, steroids decrease protein synthesis, reduce capillary sprouting, fibroblast proliferation and decrease the rate of epithelialisation.

(7) Infection – Lasting infection in wounds take place due to bacterial contamination especially when host resistance is low. Bacterial enzymes affect collagen synthesis and also delays epithelialisation. Wound haematoma, foreign bodies, overzealous diathermy, necrotic tissue, large suture ligation stumps following haemostasis act as foci for infections.

(8) Temperature of the wound – Optimum temperature for epithelial healing and other phases of wound healing is 37 degrees centigrade. Therefore use of warm saline or lukewarm water for cleansing or irrigation is of paramount importance. It is advisable never to irrigate or wash wounds with cold water.

(9) Drugs – NSAIDs, corticosteroids, and immunosuppressive drugs reduce the inflammatory process. Steroids reduce inflammation by stabilising, lysosomal membranes and also inhibit collagen synthesis. Steroids also decrease protein synthesis, capillary sprouting, fibroblast proliferation and the rate of epithelialisation. Immunosuppressive drugs interfere with mitosis (e.g. Alkylators) and protein synthesis. At the same time, immunosuppressed patients are susceptible to infections.

(10) Vitamins – Vitamin A encourages epithelialisation and formation of granulation tissue. Vitamin B Complex acts as co-factor enzymes in metabolism. Vitamin C helps in collagen synthesis and also an antioxidant. Vitamin E is also is an antioxidant.

(11) Nutrition – Malnourishment and deficiency syndrome will delay wound healing and more importantly increase the susceptibility to wound or systemic infections. Protein

deficiency is associated with reduced healing of abdominal wounds, skin, and intestinal anastomosis due to fibroblastic response reducing collagen synthesis. Nutritional deficiencies also are responsible for poor neo-angiogenesis, low collagen synthesis and wound re-modelling[11].

Zinc is an essential co-factor of enzymes activity. Copper helps in cross linkage of collagen. Iron helps to increase haemoglobin levels.

(12) Vascularity - Vascularity and high oxygen tension is important in wound healing. Facial wounds heal more quickly due to high vascularity. Good blood supply brings in oxygen, nutrients and vital cells.

(13) Surgical Technique - Poor surgical technique is responsible for poor healing. Careful attention must be given when suturing. Skin edges should very carefully apposed without any tension. Knots should not be tight to cause tattooing or ischaemia. Ugly cross-hatching sutures in exposed areas like the face should be avoided. Careless overlapping of skin prevents healing unnecessarily for months especially when applying skin clips without due care. Facial wounds number of fine proline suture can be reduced by applying paper stri-strips in between. Sutures can be removed early as 48 hours and leave steri-srips longer.

Wound dehiscence and poor anastomotic healing causes the well-known surgical disaster of anastomotic breakdown, overwhelming sepsis, systemic inflammatory response syndrome (SIRS), multi-organ failure and eventual death. If the resected end vascularity is poor and also in the presence of gross infection, it is not advisable to perform a bowel anastomosis. E.g. Diverticular perforation.

11 (*Collins C – Nutrition and wound healing 1996 : 12 (3) 87 – 90*).

Chapter 5

Types of Wounds and ulcers

Wound is a cut or break in continuity of any tissue in the body caused by injury or surgery. It describes a wide range of tissue damage.

Ulcer is defined as a break or breach in the continuity of surface epithelium, i.e. skin or mucus membrane, in various stages of healing with or without underlying tissue damage.

Surgical incisions are made with precision under strict aseptic conditions and usually bleeding is minimal or properly controlled.

Classifications of wounds According to the extent of contamination

Class I – Clean.

E.g. Elective repair of a hernia, excision of a lipoma. Antibiotics are not necessary, but when using a prosthesis, the general consensus is to use three doses of antibiotics peri-operatively.

Class II – Clean contaminated (controlled).

E.g. Cholecystectomy where bile ducts have to be divided but there is no spillage. Peri-operatively, three doses of antibiotics should be used.

Class III – Contaminated.

E.g. Spill of bile during cholecystectomy or spill of intestinal contents during bowel surgery. A minimum of five days of antibiotics are required.

Class IV – Dirty.

E.g. Diverticular perforation and faecal contamination. Prolonged intravenous antibiotics and intensive care is required.

According to its class risk of wound infection rates are 1 -2%, 6 – 9%, 13 – 20% and over 40% respectively[12].

Traumatic wounds maybe clean or dirty, tidy or untidy; cleanly cut and healthy with no tissue loss; or crushed and devitalised with tissue loss. Wounds define a wide range of damage to the body from small abrasion to extensive tissue loss.

A Classification of Wounds according to its Closure and Healing

(1) Healing by primary intention

This is also known as healing by first intention. This can occur when wound edges are brought together perfectly apposed with sutures, staples, steri-strips or glue. This is also the first intention of the surgeon and if successful, result in a cosmetically acceptable linear scar.

(2) Healing by secondary intention

These are wounds with separated edges when a large defect is made good by laying down large amounts of granulation tissues. Healing takes place base upwards and edges inwards. The important feature is wound contraction. Healing is slow and leaves a large distorted scar and is disfiguring. If the wounds are across a joint, these may cause contractions. Large wounds with skin loss, incised and drained abscesses healed in this fashion.

12(Gotttrup F Melling A Hollander D A 2005. An overview of surgical site infection aetiology, incidence and risk factors www Worldwide wounds.com 2005 E W M A Journal 2005 5 (2); 11 – 15.

(3) Delayed primary healing or healing by tertiary intention.

Here the wounds are not apposed immediately due to contamination. If the wounds are cleaned, dressed, and at a later date, edges can be excised, brought together when inflammatory and proliferative phases are well advanced. At this time some undermining of wound edges may be necessary to suture the wound without any tension.

Hypertrophic Scars

They occur soon after trauma and collagen mass remains within the bounds of the wound.

Keloid Scars

In Keloids scars collagen mass goes beyond the bounds of the wound and begins very much later in wound healing.

Types of wounds

Abrasions

Abrasions are superficial epithelial lineal scrapping. The wound is caused by frictional scrapping of skin or mucosa.

Friction Burns

Superficial epithelial scrapping of a wide area caused by friction or rubbing against an external surface.

Contusion

A bump or bruise caused by a blow or a blast. Skin maybe intact but micro or major haemorrhage in deep tissues may take place. Myofibrils of the muscles maybe damaged.

Lacerations

A torn ragged wound produced by a force that exceeds tissue strength. Avulsions, de-gloving of skin or other structures torn off its attachments off underlying tissues.

Acute wounds

Acute wounds are new wounds that heal within an expected time frame. They proceed through an orderly and timely reparative process to produce anatomic as well as functional integrity.

Wounds in trauma

AMPLE (A for Age, M for Medication, P for Past history/pregnancy, L for last meal, E for Event) The history is very important in acute injury and trauma, especially history of the event which caused the wounding.

If it is a knife wound, it is essential to know if any underlying structures are at risk, possibility of any foreign bodies, such as glass, fragments or gravel. If wounding object which has penetrated deeply or in line with vital structures such as blood vessels is still present in the wound, it should only be removed under general anaesthesia in operating theatre in a controlled manner by a surgeon.

Chronic wounds

These are wounds which failed to proceed normally through an orderly and timely reparative process. There is no time frame in which they heal. They may have arrested healing in inflammatory or proliferative phases. General consensus is that only wounds which fail to heal completely within three months is considered to be a chronic wound.

In longstanding chronic wounds, malignant transformation must be excluded.

Types of ulcers

Leg Ulcers

Most of the leg ulcers are chronic wounds. The usual causes are stasis – varicose veins, ischaemia-peripheral vascular disease, neuropathy or ischaemic neuropathy in diabetes mellitus. Other causes are infections, e.g. Tuberculosis, syphilis and also neoplasia. E.g. Squamous cell carcinoma, Basel cell carcinoma (Rodent Ulcer), Marjolins ulcer in chronic wounds and scars. Biopsy will show a histology of squamous cell carcinoma. Vasculitis also cause leg ulcers. E.g. in Rheumatoid Arthritis.

Venous Ulcers

Venous ulcers occur in areas of maximum venous hypertension or hydrostatic pressure. This occurs in the gaiter area above the malleoli where the hydrostatic pressure of the venous column is highest due to failure of unidirectional valves. Ulcers occur specially on the medial side. These are shallow and superficial ulcers and is always above the deep fascia. They have a gentle sloping edges. The floor contains granulation tissue, variable amounts of slough and exudates. Pain is usually due to tibial periostitis or gross infection.

Post thrombotic ulcers infiltrate the deep fascia and the leg has the inverted champagne bottle appearance. There are other signs of venous hypertension in the surrounding skin. They are pigmentation due to hemosiderin deposition, lipodermatosclerosis due to fat necrosis and fibrosis and atrophic blanche due to depigmentation which looks more like areas of vitiligo.

Venous hypertension is the common denominator of all sequelae of venous complications. Venous stasis is mainly due to loss of unidirectional flow towards the heart against the gravity due to incompetence of valves and failure of the calf-muscle-foot thigh pump. Joint disease, immobility, paralysis and obesity are contributing factors to the latter. Skin grafting of venous ulcer without dealing with venous hypertension is doomed to failure.

There are three theories which causes tissue damage and formation of ulcers.

(1) Fibrin Cuff Theory.

This is due to formation of proteins leaking from the capillaries forming a peri-venous infiltrate – fibrin cuff. This becomes a barrier to nutritional exchange.

(2) White Cell Trapping Theory.

White cells which adhere to the capillary wall produce cytokines which in turn cause inflammation.

(3). Chronic inflammation and Reperfusion Injury.

Inflammation due to repetitive ischaemia (during dependency and sustained venous hypertension) and reperfusion (on walking or elevation).

Ischaemic (Arterial) Ulcers

These are initially very painful, shallow non-healing ulcers with smooth margins in chronic ischaemic legs. They are usually found on the dorsum and margins of the foot, on the skin around the malleoli.

They may begin as painful erosions in between the toes. It is important for the clinicians to examine web spaces to exclude erosions and also look for fungal infections. Also feel the heel especially back of the heel for pressure sores.

Patient may also have rest pain and associated gangrene. It is important to refer all patients with rest pain to a specialist vascular surgeon to assess whether the patient is a candidate for angioplasty or revascularisation by arterial reconstruction. Sometimes these are very painful, dry deep ulcers which penetrate the deep fascia. The tendons may be exposed.

Neuropathic Ulcer and Diabetes.

Sensory loss in diabetic neuropathy characteristically has Glove and Stocking type distribution in relation to the limbs. One can use monofilament nylon thread to check the sensitivity. Neuropathy is due to demyelination of nerve fibres. This is caused by deposition of sorbitol from sugar, at the same time due to micro-angiopathy and arteriovenous shunting beneath the skin. Diabetic neuropathy may lead to a purely neuropathic foot which is warm and pulses are usually palpable. In ischaemic neuropathy the foot is cold and pulseless. It is true that diabetes goes hand in hand with atherosclerosis.

The risk areas for ulceration are on the plantar surface, underneath the first second and fifth metatarsal heads and the heel. They may form by ulceration of the skin beneath a pre-existing callosity over the bony prominences. The intervening ischemic tissues between the bone and callosity become necrotic and patient experiences pain in the callosity. Once the callosity is shaved off the ulcer underneath may reveal itself. Size of the ulcer is smaller than the callosity and may be just circular patch of unhealthy granulation tissue. There is absolutely no need to excise the whole callosity but just the small ulcer underneath.

It is important to shave off a callosity long before the pain appears. There may be embedded foreign bodies on the planter surface causing pressure necrosis. Every night before going to bed, diabetic neuropathic feet should be examined to remove any gravel, tiny stones or even dhal seeds. For shaving use of larger number 23 blade is advisable as sharp blade-edge blunts very quickly and various parts of the edge can be used.

Dorsal ulcers may develop due to pressure from footwear and they also occur on the knuckles or tips of hammer toes. Crowded footwear may cause pressure ulceration on either side of the foot. Metatarsal accommodation pads are available to lift off distal part of the metatarsal bone so that metatarsal heads are lifted off the areas of callosity.

The deformity of the foot in diabetic neuropathy is due to clawing as a result of atrophy of intrinsic muscle of the foot (Tibial nerve neuropathy) opposed by the action of powerful calf muscles acting on the foot.

Diabetes may eventually lead to Charcot's Arthroplasty casing severe deformity of the foot and pressure ulcers on the sole.

Diabetic control, regular diabetic foot care and pressure off loading by using appropriate orthotics is important, if we are to save these insensate deformed feet. Walk-in ultrasound is now available in most diabetic foot centres to detect pressure areas. Diabetes control and early shaving off, of callosities are important before necrosis of tissue takes place between it and the bone.

In established neuropathic foot, ulcers are painless and are surrounded by a rim of callosity and are the main portal of infection.

Neuro-ischaemic foot is pulseless, cold and insensate. In these patients, in addition to diabetic foot care and diabetic control, arterial reconstruction should be considered.

Tropical Ulcer (jungle rot)

As the name implies it occurs in the patients in the tropics. It is a chronic ulcerative skin lesion in the lower extremities. This start as a minor injury, abrasion or an insect bite. Ulcers are usually infected by Vincent's organisms (Borrelia Vincenti) Bacteroides and Fusiform bacteria, (fusobacterium ulcerens). Pustules may form and spread rapidly causing ulceration. The ulcer is usually round or oval in shape and has a clearly defined edge. Squamous cell carcinoma may develop with in the chronic ulcer.

Bazins Ulcer

These ulcers present in obese young females. They start as erythematous nodules (Erythrocyanosis Frigida). These maybe due to increased cold sensitivity of distal branches of the crural vessels (PTA/PA).

Martorell's Ulcer

These ulcers are common in hypertensive elderly patients. They are deep, punched out non-healing ulcers in the posterior-lateral skin of the leg. Severe pain is due to ischaemia of patches of skin due to obliteration of end arterioles.

Pressure Sores

These ulcers are very common in bed ridden patients. The main external factors are capillary occlusive external pressure over bony points and friction in moving disabled or paralysed patients in bed, without proper lifting off the bed.

Intrinsic factors are poor nutrition, anaemia, injury, infection and maceration of skin due to moisture from urine, sweat and faecal matter. Some of these patients are paralysed bed bound, sedated or unconscious. Most vulnerable areas are ischium, grater trochanter sacrum heel (calcaneus), occiput, elbows and the shin when a patient crosses their legs due to flexion contractures.

We have observed scrotal pressure sores in many bedridden patients. These occur due to friction rather than pressure. As the patient slide down scrotal sac moves under the patient causing skin damage. They are mostly grade11. Lifting the scrotal sac with Cloth Bridge on thighs is all that is required. If the patient wearing nappies best to put large gauze pack inside to lift the scrotum.

Grade   I;   Non-blanchable skin erythema.

Grade   II;   Partial thickness damage up to dermis.

Grade III; Full thickness skin damage up to subcutaneous fat, epidermis as well as dermis   destroyed.

Grade IV; full thickness skin, subcutaneous fat and fascia are damaged exposing bony points, tendons and muscles.

Pressure sore awareness;

Pressure sore awareness is vital in nursing the patient as treatment of these vulnerable patients is difficult. Two hourly turns and lifts may be the only single measure available to patients treated at home in developing countries. The pressure on the skin must be minimal and should be evenly spread at all times. Static support is given using cushions for some pressure points. These can be made of water filled disposable rubber gloves or air filled canoe shaped cushions especially for the feet. Special pressure off loading beds are now available. Water is incompressible; bodyweight therefore, spreads evenly on water mattress surface, according to Pascal's principle. Handling of water mattress is cumbersome therefore nursing homes in many countries now use air mattress.

Dynamic systems.

Dynamic alternating pressure systems e.g. water ripple beds, Quattro ripple mattresses, Nimbus Professional air mattress is unique that separate cells can be deflated and inflated for pressure off loading and wound care. Whatever the pressure, offloading devices are in dynamic modern systems, two hourly turns and lifts must still be carried out. Regardless of the mattress protection, all other devices such as water filled rubber gloves air cushions for the heels are important. Pre tibial pressure ulcers are still possible due patient crossing the legs.

Static systems.

Foams or air cushions for heels are use as static support systems. Static support systems are not as reliable as the limbs may fall off these devices. Interposing a pillow between legs will avoid pressure sores over shin.

Apart from pressure off loading, the wounds must be treated on their own merits according to its grade. Grade III or IV surgery may be required. E.g. Free tissue transfer, flap reconstruction. These should never be carried out without optimising the patient's general conditions by correcting malnutrition and anaemia as well as other factors which delays wound healing. Otherwise surgical reconstruction is doomed to failure. Post-operative care in specialised units is also important.

Chapter 6

Wound assessment.

A clinical classification for the purpose of wound assessment, treatment and selection of dressings, I have divided wounds into six groups.

(For medical students" SINGLE"– classification by Athula Withanage).

1	**S**	loughy
2	**I**	nfected
3	**N**	ecrotic
4	**G**	ranulating
5	**L**	umpy exuberant granulations(Proud Flesh)
6	**E**	pithelializing

Fig1-6.

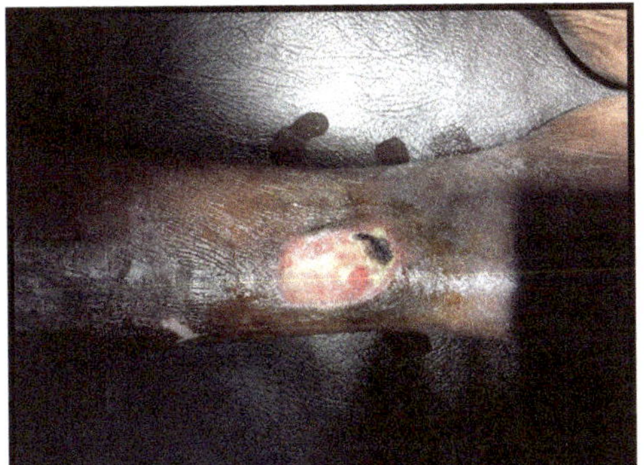

Sloughy wound

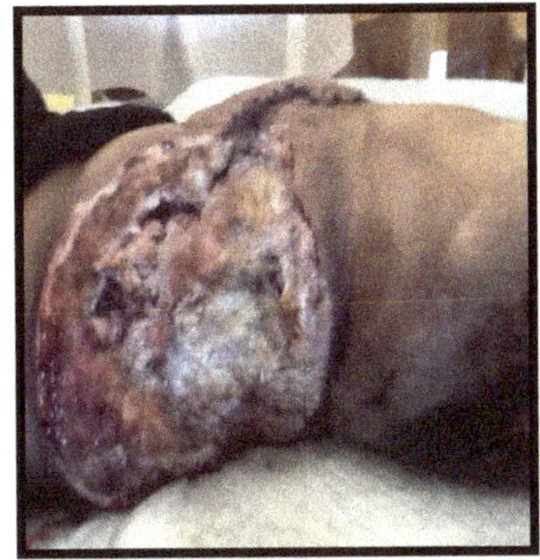

Infected wound

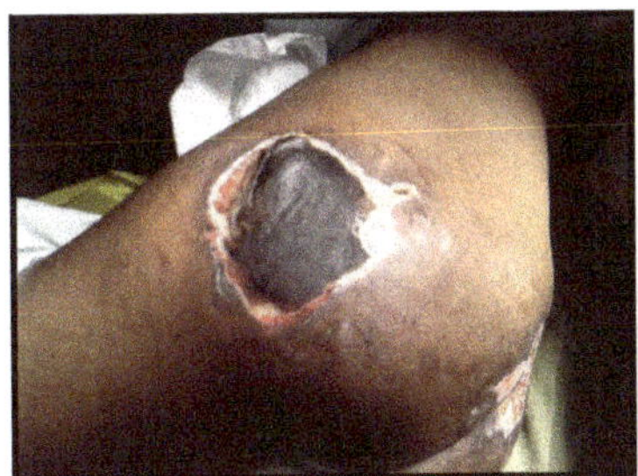

Necrotic wound

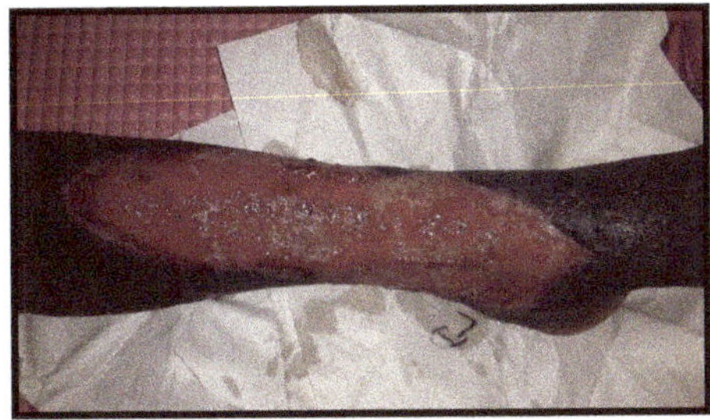

Granulating wound

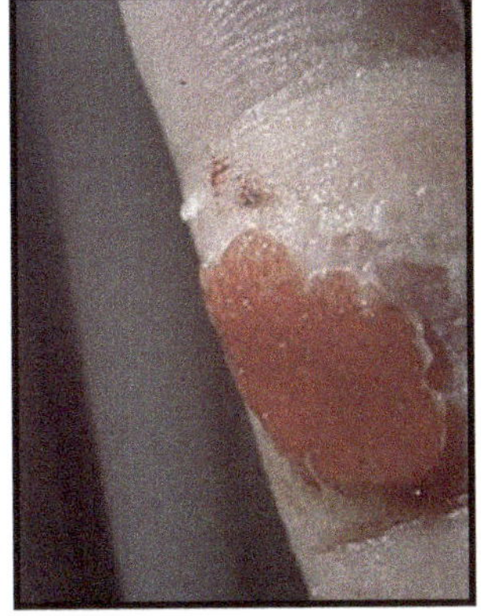

Proud flesh

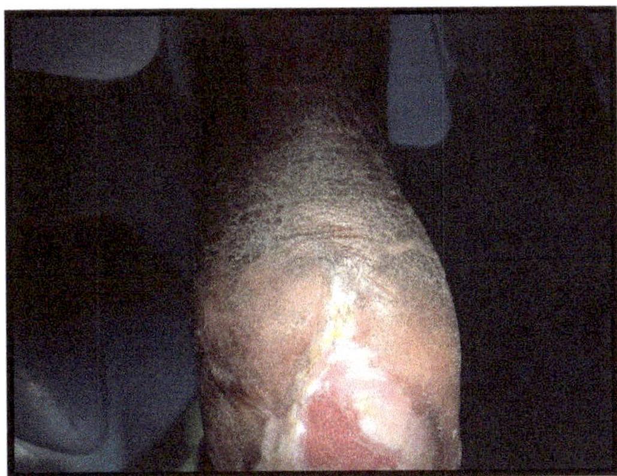

Epithelializing wound

Wound or Ulcer assessment

Description; –

1. Site –The site may point to etiological factors.

   a. Medial aspect of gaiter area - varicose ulcers
   b. Face – basal cell carcinoma
   c. Pressure points – decubitus ulcers
   d. Neck – Tuberculous, actinomycotic
   e. Feet – Ischaemic ulcers, tropic ulcers,
   f. Web spaces – Ulcers cause by fungal infections and ischaemic ulcers in diabetic feet.

2. Size – The size of the wound can be assessed by transparency films, ordinary tape measurements, Kundin Gauges, Saline moulds, Sialastic Elastomer – gives size and depth.

3. Floor – describes visible structures in the depth of the wound.

4. Base – To judge the base, the floor has to be palpated , probed and felt for fistulae, sinuses, underlying cavities and structures such as tendons, pulsation of major blood vessels, muscles, bones or bowels, foreign bodies and associated abscesses.

5. Margin – The margin of an ulcer is the line of demarcation between normal and abnormal tissues on inspection.

6. Edges – This is the part between the margin and the floor of an ulcer. The edges may indicate etiological factors.

   1. Gently sloping – healing ulcer, varicose ulcer.
   2. Undermined – Tuberculous ulcer.
   3. Raised – beaded – basal cell carcinoma.
   4. Rolled out or everted – squamous cell carcinoma

Any elevation of the edge as in 3 and 4 as well as any long standing Marjolin's type, one must consider biopsy to exclude neoplasia.

5. Punched out ulcer – decubitus ulcer, diabetic tropic ulcer, Gummatous ulcer (Syphilis)

7. Discharge –
    a. Serous discharge – varicose ulcers
    b. Blood stained discharge – chronic ulcers, malignant ulcers or freshly cleaned ulcers.
    c. Purulent discharge – This means the wound is infected.
    d. Greenish discharge – Pseudomonas infection, greenish Pyocyanin staining the dressings will eventually strike through.
    e. Yellowish discharge – this is usually due to actinomycosis discharging sulphur granules.

8. Surrounding skin (Peri-wound skin) - Classical sign of inflammation previously described maybe present around the ulcer. Spreading cellulitis and lymphangitis, skip lesions or satellite lesions may also be present. If it is a varicose ulcer, signs such as oedema, pigmentation, depigmentation (atrophie blanche), lipodermatosclerosis or large dilated tortuous feeding or draining veins maybe visible.

9. Regional Nodes – should be looked for in the drainage area of lymphatics of any ulcer. There may be simple lymphadenitis or enlarged nodes due to metastatic deposit in the node.

"The Golden Rule – The golden rule is whenever you see a lesion anywhere in the body, look for an enlarged lymph node. Whenever you find a lymph node, look for a lesion in the area of its lymph drainage"

10. Warmth of skin - It is important to check the temperature to assess inflammation or blood supply to the limb. Temperature gradient should be checked using the back of the hand from warmer thigh towards the foot. If start from the cold foot your

hand may remain cold and you may not feel the gradient. It will be high in ischaemic legs as the thigh will be warmer due to collaterals and the foot will be cold due to distal ischemia. In an ischaemic ulcer it is important to check pedal pulses and the quality of pulses can be checked with a hand held Doppler or using a colour duplex venous or arterial scan.

It is very important to assess the general condition of the patient with regard to factors influencing healing of wounds as described above.

Evaluation of the patient

Inspection of the limb involved: General appearance of the leg, such as muscle atrophy, loss of hair, dry scaly or shiny thinner pale skin, cracked deformed nails, conical shape due to loss of pulp tissue, web space fungal infections, ulcers and paronychia. All indicate chronic limb ischaemia.

Palpation: All limb pulses should be palpated with the thumb in opposition except femoral and carotid pulses. In feeling the femoral pulses one must depress the abdominal musculature around mid-inguinal point with one hand to bring the femoral artery area in to prominence. As indicated earlier, temperature gradient should be felt with the back of the hand starting from thigh (warmth) to feet (cold).

Capillary Refill - Apply pressure on the pulp of toes for 5 seconds and release. Poor vascularity is confirmed when normal pink colour does not return in 2 seconds. Venous guttering and delay in venous filling after a period of elevation are other signs of ischaemia.

Hand Held Doppler (Ultrasound probe) Examination:

A continuous US signal is transmitted from the probe and the reflected beam is picked up by a receiver in the probe. The change in frequency in the reflected beam by the moving blood cells is due to the Doppler shift. It is the frequency change that is converted to a pulsatile sound or signal. It is not the incompressible arterial wall which reflects the beam of sound.

Sometimes pressure may be high due to incompressible atheromatous arteries. In such cases retesting after exercise is important.

One must pay attention to the quality of the sounds. Tri phasic sharp sounds are considered to be absolutely normal. Bi phasic sharp sounds are also normal. Muffled monophasic sounds akin to a venous hum are indicative of poor vascularity.

Ankle Brachial Pressure Index (ABPI):

Use the sphygmomanometer and the hand held Doppler probe to measure ankle systolic blood pressure. This can be achieved even when pulse is not palpable. Brachial systolic pressure is measured in the usual manner and the best systolic pressure is obtained. ABPI is the ratio of systolic pressure at the ankle to the highest brachial systolic pressure. ABPI is normally at rest is 1. Up to 0.9 can be considered as normal. Below 0.9 to 0.7 indicates intermittent claudication. ABPI 0.5 or below indicates rest pain and patient must be referred to a vascular surgeon as soon as possible.

One must not use compression bandaging in ischemic legs especially ABPI below 0.7.

Do not use the cuff, if the leg is swollen, painful and an ulcer is present.

Duplex scanning

B mode ultra sound provides imaging of blood vessels. Doppler shift is analysed digitally by a computer. This allows detailed visualization of blood flow and the direction can be obtained. Colour duplex scanning is a useful non-invasive method available to assess vascularity of a limb but is operator dependent.

Chapter 7

Wound infections and management.

It is important to assess the bacterial burden and the need for either topical or systemic antibacterial agents.Most of the time antibiotics are not necessary unless there is associated cellulitis or generalised symptoms due to sepsis. Local application of antibiotics may cause local sensitivity reactions.

Staphylococci and Streptococci are the most common pathogenic organisms involved. Overtly infected wound with classical signs of inflammation should be swabbed and cultured. These usually have foul smelling discharge and unhealthy granulation tissues. Diagnostic yield is much better with pus or tissue than superficial swabs reflecting colonising bacteria. Pathogenic organisms invade deeper into viable tissues.

Presence of bacteria in the culture is not always synonymous with wound infections. It is important to analyse whether the wound is colonised or actually infected and if infected whether the infection is local or systemic.

Colonisation is the presence of dividing organisms within the wound. When the bio burden is increased to a critical level there maybe pain, increased discharge, malodorous exudates and unhealthy granulation tissues.

When there is local infection, classical signs of infection are present in the wound and surrounding area. When bacterial (bio) burden is over (10^5 per gm) of tissue or mm3 of pus, dividing bacteria has clearly invaded deeper viable tissue.

Contamination is the mere presence of non-replicating bacteria in the wound. Host defences i.e. immunity does not allow deeper invasion of viable tissue.

Systemic infection

Systemic dissemination of bacteria will produce generalized symptoms of sepsis. At this stage, there may be obvious regional lymphadenopathy hence the importance of examining or looking for regional nodes.

Blood culture should be taken before IV antibiotics are given, if there are rigors and spiking temperature.

Antibiotics

All infected wounds with classical signs of inflammation or patients with systemic infections need empirical systemic antibiotic treatments. If the sensitivity results of recent microbiology tests are available, appropriate antibiotics can be used. Otherwise best guess therapy can be instituted. As indicated before, cultures for antibiotics sensitivity should be taken from the wound as well as blood for culture if systemic signs and symptoms are present, prior to commencing any antibiotic treatment. In the request form, the clinician must indicate from where the cultures had been taken, time and the details of antibiotics treatment commenced or the treatment the patient may have had. The best guess antibiotic treatment will depend on the type and site of the wound.

Empirical Antibiotic Treatment (some antibiotics commonly used)

   a. Abdominal and perineal wounds; cefuroxime and metronidazole or co-amoxiclav.

b.   Diabetic foot ulcer; co-amoxiclav and ciprofloxacin.

c.   Ulcer with osteomyelitis; Co-amoxiclav and clindamycin or ciprofloxacin and clindamycin.

d.   Necrotising Fasciitis; Benzyl penicillin (high dose) and ciprofloxacin.

e.   MRSA infection; Vancomycin, Teicoplanin or Linezolid.

Once culture and sensitivity test results are available appropriate antibiotics can be given[13].

Tetanus Prophylaxis

All fresh wounds small or large should be considered at risk for development of Tetanus.

Wounds must be thoroughly cleansed and if required debrided surgically. Devitalised tissues and foreign bodies must be surgically removed.

Tetanus prone wounds;

Dirty deep wounds, puncture wounds over 1 cm in depth e.g. caused by a rusty nail, wounds contaminated with soil, manure and wounds sustained more than six hours old are prone to tetanus.

Anti-Tetanus immunisation;

a.   Immunised individuals will only require a subsequent single injection of adsorbed tetanus vaccine "Tetanus Toxoid "given intramuscularly. Tetanus vaccine (adsorbed) is a preparation of tetanus toxoid prepared by treating tetanus toxin using chemical means to render it nontoxic without losing immunogenic potency. The toxoid is then adsorbed on to a suitable adjuvant.

b.   Non immunised patients require a full course of immunisation.

13 (Brendon H Freedman A – ABC of wound healing; BMJ Vol 332 – 8 April 2006 – 838 – 839).

First injection should be followed by two more injections at six weeks and six months and a booster dose is given every ten years.

Passive immunisation is indicated with patients with tetanus prone wounds. Human Tetanus immunoglobin (HTIG) 250 units is given intramuscularly. If tetanus toxoid is given at the same time separate sites, separate limbs and separate syringes should be used.

Wound cleansing

It is well known that no wound will heal or epithelialize in the presence of necrotic tissue, slough, foreign body and infections. All wounds must be cleaned thoroughly and debrided before any forms of treatment is given.

Irrigation

1. Superficial cleansing of non-infected or colonised wounds;

Irrigation of wounds can be carried out with warm normal saline or warmed plain water. Important to check the temperature of the water by the clinician him or herself as patient may have neuropathy. Patient with normal sensation also may think it is part of the treatment and may tolerate heat for a while.

Warmth is necessary as optimum temperature for epithelial healing is 37^0C, and cold or lower temperatures slow the healing. Wounds following irrigation with cold water will take several hours to return to normal temperature.

Unnecessary and prolonged use of antiseptics such as povidone iodine (Betadine) delays healing[14].

2. Dirty infected wounds with slough

In established tissue infections (invasion of viable tissue by pathogens) antiseptics are of value.

14(Leaper D J, Simpson R A. The effect of antiseptics and topical antimicrobials on wound healing. J Antimicrobial Chemotherapy. 1986; 17 135 – 137).

Antiseptics

a. Povidone-Iodine (Betadine) - This is an inorganic disinfectant. Its halogen action is annulled by organic matter such as blood, pus and faeces. Injudicious use of betadine is detrimental, it delays wound healing in experimental animal model[15].

Betadine also can cause allergic contact dermatitis and can be absorbed systemically. Therefore it should be avoided in patients with thyroid disease and in pregnancy. It has a broader spectrum and especially significant activity against Methicillin resistant Staphylococcus aureus (MRSA). It is also available as a spray (10%, powder, cream or aqueous solution). Alcohol based solutions must not be used on open wounds, fresh or chronic. Use of Betadine is painful and also may absorbed in significant amounts.

When betadine impregnated gauze dries up in a wound, the pain may be excruciating.

b. Cetrimide (Cetavlon) 1% solution – It is a quaternary ammonium compound and has emulsifying and detergent properties. Cetrimide is moderately bactericidal, although not effective against gram negative organisms or pseudomonas. These bottles must be kept free of contamination as pseudomonas can survive in cetrimide solution. It may also be cytotoxic and may cause contact dermatitis. Cationic surface active agent of cetrimide is rapidly absorbed by fabric or gauze and gauze should not be dipped into the bottle.

c. Chlorhexidine 0.5% solution (Hibitane) - A phenolic derivative of low toxicity. Chlorhexidine is effective against Gram positive organisms. E.g. Staphylococci but not against spores.

15(Lineaweaver W. Howard R, Soucy D et al – Topical antimicrobial toxicity. Arch Surg 1085 120 ; 267 – 70.)

d. Topical antibacterials - Use of topical antibacterial in wounds are inappropriate. Resistance organisms as well as sensitivity reactions will emerge rapidly with a topical antibacterial. For bacterial colonisation simple irrigation could be sufficient. For infection if present with local signs of inflammation around the wounds, appropriate systemic antibiotics should be used.

e. Antibiotic powders which cause caking of wounds (Cicatrine, Polybactrine, Soframyacin) are now largely abandoned as the new concept of wound healing is to retain appropriate moisture within the wounds.

f. Following two antibacterial products are widely used.

1. Metronidazole gel 0.5% effectively controls smell in malodorous wounds specially caused by anaerobic bacteria [16].

2. Silver Sulphur Diazine (SSD-Flamazine) – Silver in ionic nano crystalline form had been in use for many years especially to prevent infections in severe burns. Now silver impregnated dressings are widely available and are widely used.

g. Hydrogen Peroxide - 3% or 6% solutions are useful as irrigation fluid for gritty wounds as it effervesces. It is rapidly broken down by the enzyme catalase and its antibacterial action is short lived. Hydrogen Peroxide is not active against pseudomonas. It may damage bacterial cell wall but also the normal surface skin cells (It contains catalase). Therefore, must be washed out immediately after its use.

h. Acetic Acid –2 % solution – This is effective against pseudomonas.

i. Potassium Permanganate - 0.01% solution. It is an oxidising agent. Also known as "Condys" crystals. It can be applied as a

---

16(Management of smelly tumours (editorial) Lancet 1990, 335: 141 – 42).

soaked dressing for bed ridden patients or for mobile patients as a bath in a basin. Side effects may include irritation of the skin and discolouration of clothing and skin. This is also used as a medication for a number of skin conditions such as fungal infections, impetigo, pemphigus, dermatitis and tropical ulcers. For tropical ulcers it is used with procaine benzyl penicillin.

Methicillin Resistant Staphylococcus aureus (MRSA)

Some strains of Staphylococcus aureus became resistant to penicillin/methicillins over time and are difficult to treat since they are resistant to all beta lactam antibiotics. MRSA infections were common in hospitalized patients but now even community acquired cases are also increasing in number.

Risk factors

Prolong hospital stay

Immunocompromised

Recent antibiotic therapy

Wounds/IV lines

In the community
   waxing or tattooing procedures, contact with MRSA infected patient, prisoners and military personnel

Management

Barrier nursing
Isolation from other patients to prevent spread of infection
Standard precautions when dressing and handling of these patients
Chlorhexidine wash/bath daily (0.25-2%)
Antibiotics according to culture and sensitivity
Rotational antiseptic dressings
May need wound cleaning

Pseudomonas wound infection

Pseudomonas aeruginosa is the other common organism isolated from chronic wounds other than Staphylococcus aureus. It has both intrinsic and acquired antibiotic resistance making wound management challenging. It can even grow in wounds which are dressed with povidone iodine, chlorhexidine and savlon
It can be found in Respiratory tract, blood, CNS, heart, GI/GU tract and skin.
Greenish colour of pus or wound tissue or the overlying dressing indicates pseudomonas infection.

Management

Drying kills bacteria. Pseudomonas loves moisture
Standard precautions when dressing and handing of these patients
Antiseptic wash daily/Bath
Antibiotics are used according to C+S
Wound cleansing - Chronic wounds – leg ulcers;

Pre Hospital Phase; Patients are advised to have warm tap water shower and wrap the affected parts with clean or if available sterile paper before coming to hospital for dressings. It may be possible to provide these sterile dressing packs after the each visit. Forceful direct washing of the wound should be avoided as some wounds may bleed. Gentle sideways wash with trickling water is sufficient.

For any bleeding varicose ulcer, the limb should be bandaged, with the leg well elevated by another person, with veins empty from toes upwards.

Hospital Phase; Initially warm tap water or warmed saline (bags can be dipped in warm water) can be used as irrigation solution. Cold fluids slow down healing and the wound remain cold for some time and will contribute to poor healing.

For dirty infected wounds, antiseptics such as chlorhexidine, cetrimide or betadine can be used but it should be kept in mind that some are inactivated by the presence of blood and pus. Cetrimide and betadine are cytotoxic against fibroblasts. Hydrogen peroxide is a natural disinfectant and bacteria are instantly killed but it is important to remember it kills normal cells as well and disrupts the cellular integrity of tissues. It can be used to cleanse the wounds. The wound should be thoroughly washed after its use.

In short most substances used for cleansing should be washed away before applying the definitive dressing.

Wound Malodour control.

Malodour is a result of bacterial activity and due to accumulation of short and medium chain volatile fatty acids.

1. **Metrotop / Metrogyl** - It is a hypromellose gel containing 0.8% v/v Metronidazole BP and Benzalkonium chloride solution BP 0.02% v/v. Ideal to combat infection in malodorous wounds. Gel combat the odour produced by the bacteria and is effective not only against anaerobes but also act on volatile fatty acids (VFA).

2. **Activated charcoal dressings** – These absorb toxins, bacterial spores and pro inflammatory proteases. Malodorous molecules are attracted to the surface of the carbon and adsorbed by an electrostatic mechanism[17]

Indications are fungating, discharging and malodorous acute or chronic wounds. Charcoal dressings are not indicated for dry wounds.'

Antibacterial agent like silver can be added to these dressings.

Other Dressings available for malodorous wounds.

17Thomas.S,Fisher.B,Fram.P.J,Waring.M.J, ; Odour absorbing dressing. J.of wound care 1998 7; 5. 246-250.

1. Actisorb silver. - Activated charcoal dressing impregnated with silver.

2. Sorbsan plus carbon – non adhesive calcium alginate fibre pad with absorbent viscose backing containing activated charcoal. Good for malodourous heavily exuding wounds

Burns

In adults the surface area loss is calculated by Wallace's rule of nine. Patient's palmer surface of the hand as well as genitalia is equal to 1% each. In children the head represent a large area than in adults. Intravenous fluid replacement is vital for children over 10% surface area of burns, and adults over 15%,. Obviously these patients need hospital admission. Patients should be catheterised and hourly urine output must be accurately measured. All patients with non-accidental burns or injuries must be admitted to hospital and appropriate referrals must be made.

1. Partial thickness burns

a. First degree burns. E.g. sun burns.-

There is severe pain and erythema but initially there are no blisters. Surface does blanch on pressure. Germinal epithelial layer is intact.

b. Second degree burns –

the skin is painful and oedematous and the surface is wet with blister formation. Elements of germinal epithelial layer remains.

2. Full thickness Burns (Third degree.)

This is also known as third degree burns and appears dark, leathery, mottled and waxy-white. The surface is painless, but the edges are still painful. These patients as well as patients with facial burns suspected of inhalational injury must be treated in the burns unit with intensive care facilities. Cough, shortness of breath, hoarseness, noisy breathing, red eyes, soot in saliva, carbonaceous sputum, singeing of the eyebrows, eye lashes and nasal vibrissae, facial burns, neck swelling are the tell-tale signs of an inhalational injury. If one has to transfer the patient to a burns unit pre-emptive endotracheal intubation may be required.

All children with suspected non-accidental burn injury (NAI) must be admitted to the hospital. This should be carried out very diplomatically until NAI is confirmed.

Treatment begins with primary survey – (A B C D E protocol of ATLS) and stabilisation of the patient. For fluid resuscitation, estimation of burnt body surface area (second and third degree) and the weight of the patient is required. In addition to intravenous fluid resuscitation the patients with inhalation injury should be carefully watched. Carboxyhaemoglobin levels in blood may rise to a level of 10%. Monitoring of hourly urine output is essential.

Clothes soaked in chemicals must be removed without further damaging the skin. If necessary clothes should be cut out. Dry chemical powder should be brushed off from the skin and clothes first. Then chemicals should be flushed away with a large amount of cool water using a gentle flowing water. Hard sprays or jets should not be used.

Eyes should be irrigated immediately after injury with water. Eyes should be irrigated in medical care centres with using normal saline or sterile water until conjunctival cul-de-sac ph. Is below 8 for alkali burns. If not must continue with intermittent irrigation and litmus tests. It will be helpful to use a topical anaesthetic and lid speculum.

In skin burns acids should be washed for ½ hour. The damage is usually kept limited to the area of contact and does not usually cause damage deep in the tissues. Alkaline burns must be washed for a minimum of 60 min as they penetrate deeply than acids. Begin rinsing immediately as this can reduce complications. If there is still a burning sensation continue rinsing for a further period. Treatment of chemical burns never involves neutralization of acid or base as the resultant exothermic reaction worsens tissue injury. Alkali burns can progress to full thickness rapidly cause saponification of fat cells and cause liquefaction necrosis. Unattached alkali molecules then are free to penetrate deeper.

Acid hydrolyses proteins soon after contact causing coagulative necrosis forming a tough lathery eschar which limits further penetration.

Infuse fluids to produce at least 1ml of urine per kg in children weighing less than 30 Kgs and 0.5 ml of urine in adults.

Surface area is calculated only for second and third degree burns. The rate given is 4 ml per Kg per 24 hours (4xKgsxTBSA %) half the calculated dose is given during the first 8 hours after the burn injury and the rest over the next 16 hours (Parkland-Baxter formula). This is because gross hypovolaemia is due to maximum fluid loss during the first 8 hours.

It is important to remove all jewellery, especially from digits. If it is already swollen due to the burn some of the jewellery should be removed by cutting. For circumferential burns, surgical incision up to bleeding tissues (escharotomy) will be required under general anaesthesia. Fasciotomy may be required in some cases. If the burn surface area is more than 20%, nasogastric tube aspiration is required. After initial washing with sterile saline and 1% chlorohexidine, the dead tissue can be removed under general anaesthesia. Small blisters can be left intact. Large blisters which will eventually burst spontaneously should be aspirated under sterile condition with a needle and a syringe. The epithelial covering of the blister can be temporarily pressed back into place.

Tetanus immunisation and antibiotics are also important in burns.

Electrical Burns

Body is a volume conductor of electrical energy. Clinically skin maybe spared but the deep muscle maybe necrotic. Rhabdomyolysis results in myoglobin release causing acute renal failure. The urine itself maybe dark with haemochromogens. If myoglobinuria is present it is important to make sure urine output is over 100 ml/hour. Mannitol and bicarbonate can be given as myoglobin dissolves in alkaline urine.

Chapter 8

Modern concept of wound healing

"Moist Wound Healing "

Zoologist George Winter (1927 – 1981) introduced the modern concept of "moist wound healing" in 1962. In a study published in Nature in 1962 he demonstrated that epithelialisation occurred twice as faster in moist wounds than in the wounds which were kept dry sometimes with a large dry scab.

His experiments on pigs proved that epidermal migration is much faster in moist wounds. Since then other authors have proved the benefits of moist wound healing. A moist environment also has a role in the debridement of devitalised tissues.

Appropriate moisture in the wound environment helps to rehydrate and autolyse dead tissues. Autolytic wound debridement can be achieved by using gel formers such as Carboxy-Methyl Cellulose (CMC), Pectin or Gelatine. Gel-formers will rehydrate, soften and autolyse necrotic tissue and provide a moist environment promoting granulation tissue formation and epithelialisation.

Old concept of encouraging drying up of wounds and encouraging scab formation has now been largely abandoned. Patients still do request medications or dressings to "dry up the wound". So often what they mean are antibiotics.

Moist wound healing may not be appropriate for some wounds such as necrotic digits in diabetic patients, as infection is a greater risk. In this situation the wounds are not expected to heal until auto amputation of necrotic digit or gangrenous skin takes place

In order to maintain the appropriate moisture in a wound treated with gel formers, vapour permeable, bacterial occlusive, self-adhesive, polyurethane, foam dressings are used as secondary wound dressings.

Chapter 9

Management of painful wounds

Management of pain in wounds especially in extensive wounds like burns require a thoughtful humane approach. Pain is not inevitable in wound care.

There are three types of wound pain in wound management

- Pain experienced while the dressing is in place

- Pain caused during cleansing or debridement

- Pain during the change of wound dressing

Staff must take all possible measures to minimise the pain associated with wound management. Superficial "skin pain" is described as "cutting or burning". Deeper wounds cause throbbing and if nerve endings are involved as stinging or tingling. One of the main causes of pain is stimulation of nerve endings by local dehydration. This occurs every time slap in betadine dressing is applied to every wound which will eventually dry up.

The modern concept of wound healing is therefore, maintaining a moist interface does help in pain control as well as healing.

Emotional Scars;

Wounds especially chronic wounds, will inevitably leave emotional as well as physical scars. They are often impossible to detect. Wounds may heal but emotional scars may remain. Coming to terms with loss of bodily functions or altered body image is often difficult.

Emotional responses include fear about the future, frustration due to poor progress in wound healing, overwhelming smell, loss of physical capacity, anxiety, loss of self-esteem, vulnerability by being helpless, depression and sense of worthlessness.

Family members, medical staff, carers who genuinely make an effect to understand patients can help the patient to cope with these problems. Religious faith is also important. Most of all, a wound care specialist must take greater care and interest in patients and must institute correct wound care and build up hope to the suffering patient.

EMBRACE HOPE – WOUNDS ARE CURABLE.

Altered body image

How the patient feel about his or her body and appearance may result in depression. These are due to lack of self-esteem, sexual problems and guilt about the responsibility of their own condition.

The patient must be encouraged to talk about his or her own illness. The care giver must listen carefully to what the patient has to say and help them to come to terms with their physical as well as emotional scars.

Introverted behaviour is common due to depression, due to denial and anger. The patients must be helped to adjust to the new reality, e.g. loss of limb or any organ (e.g. breast.) It is also possible to overcome the disability and rehabilitate the patient by offering various appliances and reconstructions. It is important to support the family members who volunteer to offer care for the patient as the impact to the family also may be devastating. For E.g.: Some of our patients thought that they would have a hole in the chest wall for ever following mastectomy. Therefore informed consent and counselling by the clinician and breast care nurse is of paramount importance.

Chapter 10

Basic Concepts Of Wound Dressings

Ambrose Pare (1500)

Je le pansai et Dieu le guerit.

I closed it, god healed it.

Ambrose Pare (1510-1590) was a French barber surgeon who noticed the popularised mystique of wound healing. He was the father of haemostasis by ligation. In 1522, near Metz in France, he bandaged a man with 12 sword wounds. To everyone's surprise he recovered. In treating battle field wounds, this is the philosophy he used throughout his career. This is now an ineradicable art of surgical heritage. Although he thought occlusion was the treatment, experimenting on various types of dressings (rose oil, egg yolk, turpentine), he discovered that what you dress the wound with, does matter.

At present in most developing countries wounds are dressed with betadine impregnated gauze. Firstly injudicious use of betadine delays wound healing. When the wound dries up it causes excruciating pain to the patient by stimulation of nerve endings due to local drying up of tissues.

Locally made gauze which are cut and stitched in hospitals before sterilisation does leave fragments of gauze material in the wound causing foreign body reaction and infection. Packing the wound cavities with gauze will leave many fragments and it will result in chronic abscess cavities E.g. laid open Pilonidal abscess cavities

Dressing should fit the phase of healing, type and state of the wounds and should create an ideal wound environment with appropriate moisture as described by George Winter (1962).

Appropriate wound dressings need to be selected based upon holistic assessment of both the patient and the wound. This approach may help to promote healing and reduce healing times.

In treating any wound, control of exudate and protection of peri-wound skin is vital. For this maintaining appropriate moisture in the wound bed is important. If there is sensitivity reaction a low percentage steroid ointment can be used. E.g. 0.1% dexamethasone.

The selection of a wound dressing is dependent on the assessment of the patient's wound including stages of wound healing, exudate levels, the surrounding skin, patient sensitivities and patient choice. Exudate level will indicate as to what absorbency that the dressing should possess. Management of the exudate effectively will prevent maceration and excoriation of the peri-wound skin. The key to effective skin protection is the use of barrier products that are non-sensitizing and do not leave a sticky residue. There are gels ointments, touch free sprays and pastes available in the market based on demithicone, petrolatum, Manuka honey and Zinc oxide. 10% zinc oxide paste is perhaps the most popular in developing countries.

A dressing requires changing when there is "strike through" i.e. the exudate is coming through the dressing, the outside of the dressing is wet or it is leaking.

All wound care specialists must have some knowledge in vascular assessment of limbs especially the lower limbs. This is important especially when applying compression bandages or stockings.

Chapter 11

Choosing an appropriate wound dressing

Choosing a wound dressing should be carried out based on common wound characteristics. All dressings should be appropriate moisture retentive as the latter is the modern concept of wound healing. Wound assessment is very important to determine whether the wound is acute or chronic, stage of healing, how much exudate the wound is producing etc. chronic wounds may get stuck in one of the phases of wound healing (inflammatory, proliferative or remodelling), mostly in the inflammatory phase.

One must also remember that uncontrolled matrix metalloproteinases are a major underlying cause for chronicity. Dressings should optimize the healing process in each stage and should be cost effective. In cooperation of antimicrobial agents in the dressing, will help to target and kill bacteria. Choosing the correct dressing decreases time to healing and improves patient quality of life. Practitioner's main aim should be as follows;

1. Promote and support natural healing process.

2. Create and maintain an ideal wound environment – A moist wound healing environment: concept promoted by George Winter[18].

3. Prevent secondary damage as well as iatrogenic damage caused

18(Winter G D formation of scab and rate of epithelisation of superficial wounds in the shin of the young domestic pig. Nature 1962; 193: 293 – 294)

by materials used for dressings and injudicious inappropriate dressing change.

4. Irrigate the wound with appropriate warm solutions and avoid cold lavage which will delay healing.

5. Use an ideal dressing which is non-irritant, non-allergenic and atraumatic. It is important to get a proper history in relation to previous treatment and dressings.

6. Evaluate, plan and implement wound care with consideration for the individual patient and not just the wound. To do this, it is of paramount importance to assess aetiological factors, other co-morbidities and patient's social background. While treating the wound, etiological factors must be dealt with such as control of diabetes, revascularisation of the leg and treatment of venous stasis and venous hypertension (varicose veins).

7. Give care and attention to social and psycho-sexual problems, associated with wounds on the face, neck, breast, abdomen and genitalia.

8. Maintain privacy and confidentiality, respect patient's culture, religious beliefs and patient's choice.

Types of dressings available.

1. Semi permeable film dressings.

(Permeable to air & vapour, impermeable to liquids and bacteria)

These allow the wounds to breathe as they are permeable to water vapour and air. Impermeability to liquids and bacteria helps to maintain a moist environment and prevents contamination from exterior.

At the same time patient can have a shower without contamination. Moisture levels are determined by the moisture vapour transmission rate (MVTR). Semi permeable films are very thin polyurethane cling like films coated with acrylic adhesive. They come with backing sheets or frame work to facilitate applications to prevent wrinkling adhering to it and gloves.

As these are transparent, clinician can inspect the wound for collections, haematoma and infection without disturbing the process of healing. Peri wound skin contact should be at least 4 cm from the edge of the wound for adequate adherence. These can be only used on wounds with minimal or no exudate. Films are not absorptive and peri wound may macerate if exudate is allowed to collect here. For the same reason these films are not suitable for infected exuding wounds. [19]

Indications;

1. Post-operative incisional class 1 wounds.
2. Wounds with subcuticular sutures.
3. Superficial minor burns.
4. Grazes
5. Skin graft harvesting donor sites.
6. Dressing over joints and creases. Edges can be snipped to fit the curvatures.
7. IV catheter or cannula sites. Special readymade dressing available with a base for this purpose.

Examples are;

Hydrofilm, Opsite, Mepore.

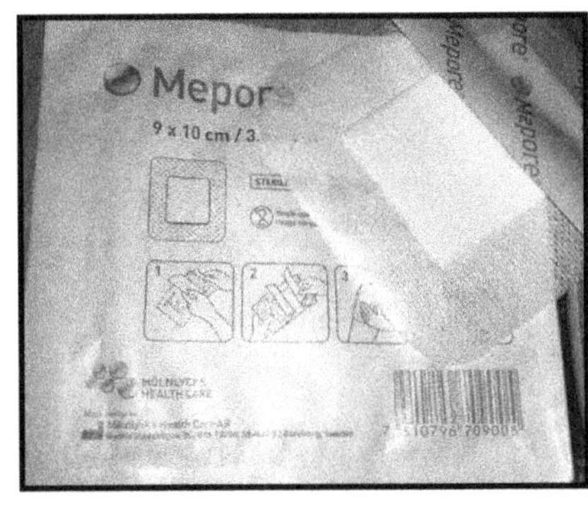

[19] G. Dabiri, E.Damstetter, T.Phillips Choosing a wound dressing based on common wound characteristics. Advanced .Wound care2016 Jan 1; 5(1); 32-41.

2. Absorbent Dressings;

(Island sheet [absorbent] dressings)

These can be used on wounds where mild absorbency of exudate is required or on wounds where slight ooze of blood or uninfected exudate is expected. Ideal for post-operative sutured or clipped (Stapled) incisions. These consist of an island sheet of absorbent soft viscose, polyester bonded pad backed with a shower proof adhesive hypoallergenic border. Absorbency increases with the increasing thickness of the absorbent (Sheet) layer. They are permeable dressings that allow moisture absorbed from the wound to evaporate.

These are called "Island dressings". They come in a frame delivery system. Thicker dressings are more absorbent and can be used in chronic wound as a secondary dressing. These dressings are not suitable if the exudate is relatively thick, also not for heavily bleeding or oozing wounds.

Heavily exuding wounds produces over 5 ml of exudate per 10 cm2 per 24 hours.

Indications

Primarily closed post-operative wounds, sutured or clipped with perfect apposition. .

Protection for primarily sutured or clipped clean post-operative acute wounds with significant depths

1 Laparotomy wounds.
2 Sternotomy wounds.

E.g. Medipore plus pad, Opsite Plus, Opsite post op, Primapore, Tegaderm plus Pad. Telfa, tegaderm plus pad, Melolin.

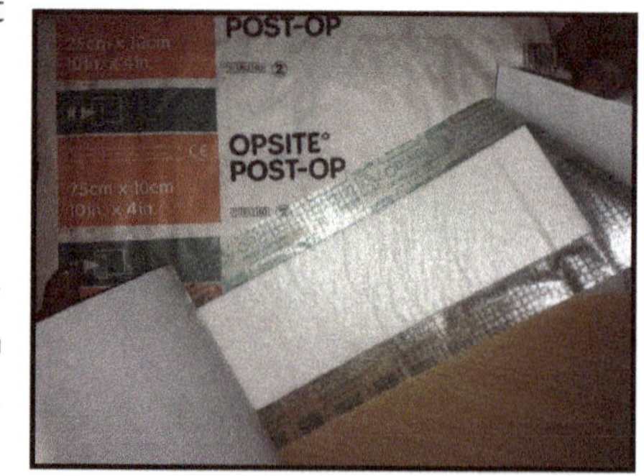

3. Hydrocolloids.

The most modern dressing developed since the Winter's concept of modern wound care to provide a moist wound environment. Hydrocolloids are biodegradable.

They are composed of Carboxy-Methyl Cellulose (CMC), a synthetic cellulose derivative, the principal gel forming agent.

Some dressings such as Granuflex contain gelatin, pectin and also other elastomeric polymers and adhesives. Most of these are gel formers. They absorb water from exudate and swell. The adhesive layer forms a cohesive gel when in contact with wound exudate.

Main value is in the treatment of wounds containing slough and necrotic tissue.

Granulation tissue formation and epithelialisation cannot take place as long as slough and necrotic tissue remains in the wound.

1. Duoderm; Duoderm sheet is thinner than others, prevents loss of water vapour and rehydrates the dead tissue which is then removed by autolysis with the removal of the dressing.

2. Granuflex; Granuflex sheet has an outer layer of polyurethane foam film.

3. Dressings like Comfeel sheet has a vapour permeable film backing, bevelled edges to reduce the risk of rucking.

Therefore these dressings should be used on dry necrotic tissue but should not be used on muscle and bone and in heavily exuding wounds. All are impermeable to exudate and microorganisms.

Minimum overlap of 2 cm from the wound margin is required. If there is no exudate the dressings can be left for five to seven days. Some are designed to be in place for up to a week. These dressings are expensive and should be left for a minimum of 5 days and another advantage of these "stick on "or" slapped on "dressing is that the sheet can be partially lifted to see the state of autolysis or the presence of any infection in the wound.

Indications for hydrocolloid dressing,

Dry necrotic wounds or lightly exuding wounds

Pressure sores stage 1 & 2. E.g. Granuflex has cross linked adhesives with the gel formers are ideally suited for early pressure sores. They can be used as a "slapped on" dressing on the necrotic dry skin. Ideal for back of the heel grade1 pressure sore. Where ever a non-blanchable patch on skin is seen, this is the best dressing. It can be lifted to see whether damage has progressed or healed. Pressure off loading still should not be forgotten.

1. On skin vulnerable to friction to prevent stage 1 bedsores converting to stage 2. E.g. non-blanchable bedsores grade 1, such as back of the heel, elbows and shin areas.

2. Minor superficial partial thickness burns.

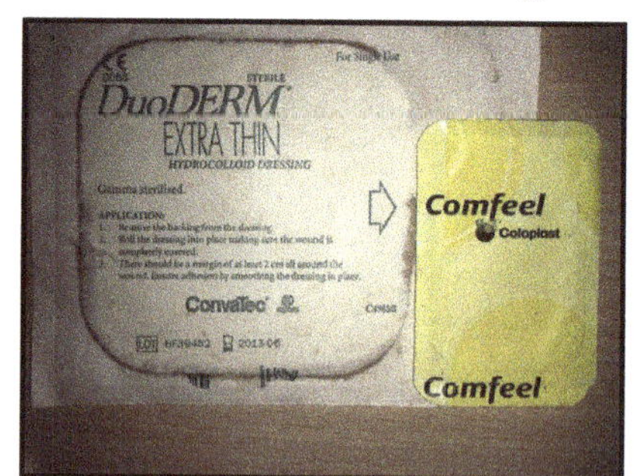

3. Skin donor sites

4. Abrasions.

As these dressings are expensive they must be applied *on wounds less than 0.5% BSA only*

4. Hydro Gels.

(Always applied with a gel retaining secondary dressing)

They were the first biomaterials developed for human use. It is a macro molecular polymer gel constructed on a network of cross linked polymer chains and has the ability to absorb large amount of fluid via hydrogen bonding.

Therefore hydrogels provide an ideal moist wound environment. They will require a secondary dressing because of the amorphous shapeless nature of the gel. These are soothing and cooling dressings, comfortable and easy to use. Dressing change is relatively painless.

It is important to remember that drying out betadine gauze packs widely used in developing countries are agonizingly painful and delays healing. Hence the knowledge about these wound dressing products are very important to any practitioner.

Hydrogels are ideally suited to the management of dry gangrenous patches of skin and wounds forming leathery eschar. It contains 90% water but softening or autolytic debridement will best take place with some proteolytic enzymes of the exudate.

Hydrogels rehydrate, soften and facilitate autolysis. Scoring or surface cross hatching of the necrotic patch can be carried out painlessly to facilitate the rehydration.

The following few points are very important in using hydrogel and preparation of the wound.

1. In a dark skinned person sensory test should be carried out before cross hatching to determine the viability of the skin. Skin may be merely darkened by use of Condys water or may be the patient's real colour of the skin. Following application of hydrogel, a containing secondary dressing such as a semipermeable dressing should be applied.

2. Propylene glycol a constituent of hydrogel is toxic to larvae of maggots and must be thoroughly washed before maggot therapy.

3. Hydrogel may create a condition ideal for the survival of anaerobic bacteria and should be used with a caution. Perhaps it is best not to use hydrogels in infected wounds, third degree burns and profusely excluding wounds.

4. As hydrogel partially hydrated it can also be used in moist wet conditions. It is important to watch for maceration of periwound skin.

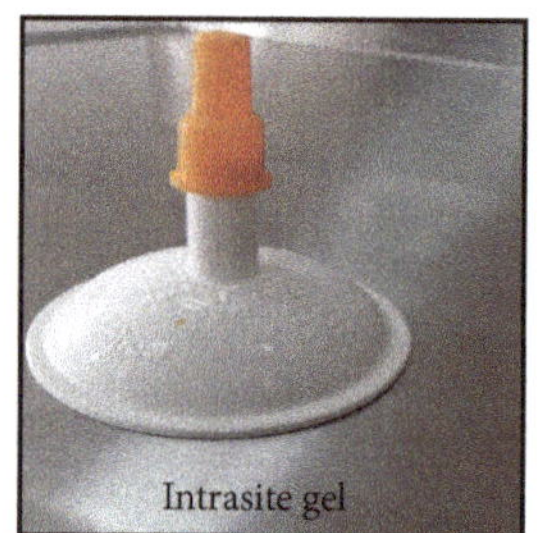

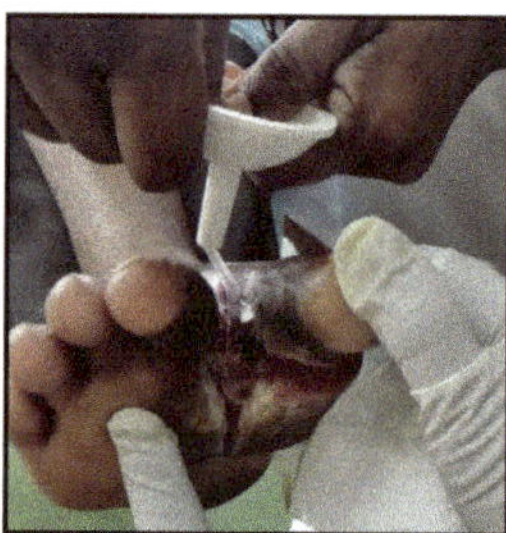

E.g.:- Intrasite gel, Suprasorb G Gel, Hydrosorb gel

Remember hydrogels kill maggots and may create an anaerobic conditions.

These are not hydrocolloids but have similar properties. As indicated above, all need a secondary dressing.

Gel sheets;

Hydrosorb Comfort, Actiform cool are hydrogel sheets which will either hydrate or donate fluid depending on the amount of moisture in the wound.

Moisture promotes granulation tissue formation and at the same time the high water content debrides necrosis.

5. Alginates. (For wounds with moderate to large amount of exudate, best for slightly deeper wounds and exudate must be present for gelling)

Alginates are derived from brown seaweed Phaeophyceae. They are highly absorbent and biodegradable. They consist of calcium or sodium salts of alginic acid and are available in the form of sheets or ropes. There are two types of alginic acids.

A soft flexible gel is formed if Mannuronic acid predominates e.g. Sorbsan. This gel is soft and can be easily irrigated off the wound or cavity.

A firmer gel is formed slowly if Guluronic acid predominates e.g. Kaltostat. As the dressing maintains its form it can be easily removed en-block.

Dressing change in both is smooth, atraumatic and painless. Alginate ropes or sheets can absorb 20 times their own weight in fluid and can be used in wounds that produce moderate to large volume of exudate.

Alginate dressing always requires a secondary dressing.

Over enthusiastic compression may reduce absorbency. Not suitable for dry necrotic wounds as gelling will not occur without exudate.

Indications;

1. Leg ulcers

2. Cavity wounds

3. Pressure sores

4   Wide mouth sinuses. Use in small mouthed sinuses may prevent drainage as the tract becomes blocked with the alginate plug especially those containing Guluronic acid forming a firmer gel.

Change the dressing when the secondary dressing has reached its absorbent capacity. Do not let the exudate seep through or strike through. Any dressing must be changed when outer bandage is soaked i.e. strike through. It does not matter even if it happens a few hours after the dressing was done. It may be possible that the selection of the dressing for that particular wound is not correct.

Alginates ropes are useful for haemorrhagic cavities following incision and drainage of abscesses such as peri-anal, pilonidal or ischio-rectal. Calcium alginates have haemostatic properties due to the fact that calcium is released in exchange for sodium in the exudate when alginate comes in contact with the latter. Released calcium ions activate platelets.

Alginate sheets are ideal for painful skin graft donor sites on the thigh.

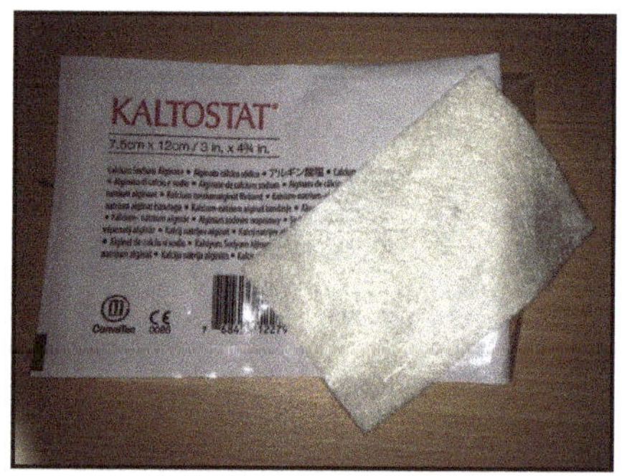

Examples of alginates ;

Sorbsan can be left to lie over the edge of the wound

Kaltostat should be trimmed to fit.

6. Foams. (Absorbent & super absorbent with a water repellent outer layer).

Foams come in two forms, either polyurethane or silicone. Some need a secondary dressing, others are self-adherent. Foaming the polymer produces cells within and provides it with absorbent or superabsorbent properties. Standard thicknesses of form sheets are 4mm to 7mm but extra thin sheets are available at 1 mm thickness.

They have an outer covering of a transparent film which is water repellent. It provides a water repellent barrier property and prevents strike through.

Foam chips in a polymeric envelope can be used for cavity wound dressings. It is an innovative moisture control layer that allows the dressing to effectively respond to changing exudate levels within the wound.

These dressings are suitable for moderately exuding wounds. They should not be used on dry wounds or eschars. They can be used as a secondary dressing over hydrogels. They can be used for over 7 days or until strike through occurs from sides. Their fluid handling capacity depends on thickness, absorbency and Moisture Vapour Transmission Rate (MVTR).

Silicone foam dressing is formed by polymers of silicone elastomer. The foam is produced by mixing base liquid and catalyst. The chemical reaction produces some heat but sensation is not troublesome. As the soft foam is formed the dressing conforms to the precise contours of the cavity or wound. Therefore ideal for electively laid-open pilonidal cavity after the haemostatic alginate for 48 hours.

Excellent for pilonidal cavity laid open surgically in the natal cleft but retaining is difficult without a suitable secondary dressing.

e.g. Allevyn Adhesive, Lyoform (non-adhesive).

Indications.

1. Mild or moderately exuding ulcers

2. Post op wounds.

3. Pilonidal cavity wounds (especially silicone elastomer)

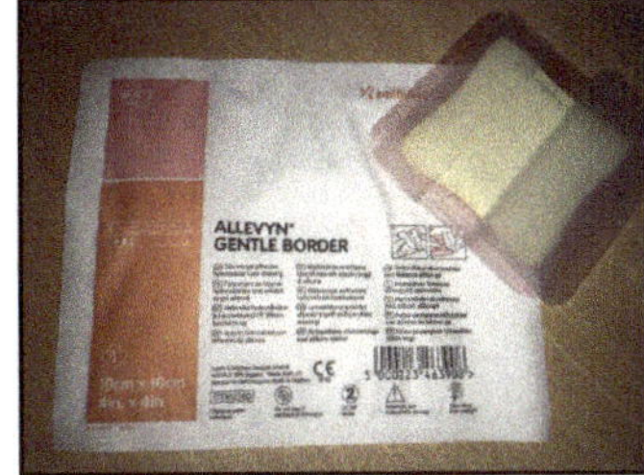

4. 3rd degree burns.

5. Pressure sores.

6. Tie over, over skin grafted ulcers

7. Rapid capillary action dressings.

1. This is a three layer dressing designed to rapidly absorb exudates and interstitial fluids and optimize condition for healing at the wound-dressing inter phase (Winter's moist healing environment). They are made from a triple layer of polyester and viscose fibre (Advadraw) with a perforated wound contact polymer film to prevent adhesion to granulation tissue. The fluid will be transferred from one layer to the other in a methodical way. The dressing can be easily cut to the shape of the wound. Fluid is drawn vertically in to the dressing and there is no lateral movement at the wound interphase which could cause maceration of the periwound skin.

Spiral presentation is also available for deeper cavities and sinus tract while mouth of the tract can be covered with layered version. Do not cut the spiral ribbon as fibre may leave fragments in the wound.

These are not Gel formers and can be removed in one piece. Subsequent irrigation also may not be necessary.

These dressings are most effective for sloughy highly exuding wounds.

2. Bio ceramic Microporous Alumina Sphere Dressings; this is also a capillary force driven absorption dressing (e.g. CERDAK). Alumina (aluminium oxide) sphere granules are in a sachet made of non-woven fabric. Suction power of alumina sphere siphons out excess wound exudate. Must not cut the sachets for any reason. Porosity within the sachet is 75% and atmospheric oxygen can circulate in interstices. There is no continuous liquid phase between trapped within and fresh wound exudate. Here

there is two to four fold activity of growth enhancing proteins , especially the enzymes;

a. Histidine decarboxylase.

b. Ornithine decarboxylase.

c. Amino acid hydroxyprolene.

As it is not a gel former for moderately exuding wound I use fine layer of intrasite gel as a primary dressing and Alumina sphere dressing as secondary dressing. This may be controversial.

8. Honey - Medical Grade;

Honey contain 80% of sugar and 17% of water. Medical grade honey is filtered of impurities, gamma radiated and produced under sterile hygienic conditions.

It is a potent antibacterial agent and therefore can be used in infected wounds. It should be undiluted to retain its antibacterial property. It should be used in minimum or moderately oozing wounds as excessive exudate dilutes the honey. In diabetics it can be used with blood sugar monitoring.

Manuka honey is also known as the best natural antibiotic of the world. Honey is active against Pseudomonas aeruginosa, MRSA, Vancomycin Resistant Enterococcus (VRE) and other multi resistant organisms. There is no evidence of bacterial resistance.

Honey

1. Causes autolytic debridement.
2. Reduce inflammatory activity.
3. Reduce oedema of underlying tissues by drawing of fluid by osmosis.
4. Stimulates granulation tissue formation.

5. Reduces inflammation and oedema

6. Reduces pain.

7. It has antibacterial activity.(see above)

Contra indication is known allergy to bee venom. Protect peri-wound skin from maceration using a secondary dressing.

E.g.Activon Honey. Medical grade Menuka honey. Honey impregnated tulle is also available.

Indications.

1. Infected wounds and ulcers.

2. Foul smelling wounds as honey deodorizes. Bacteria prefer sugar to amino acids which produces malodorous compounds.

3. Granulating wounds.

4. Pressure sores

5. Burns

6. Graft sites.

7. Dry or sloughy necrotic wounds.

9. Antimicrobials.

Only a few antibiotics are recommended for topical use because of sensitization and development of bacterial resistance.

Eg:-

1. Metronidazole

2. Mupirocin

3. Sulphadiazine (sulphonamide) in silver sulphadiazine(SSD)

4. Soframycin (framycetin) sofra-tulle dressing. Fusidinetulle.

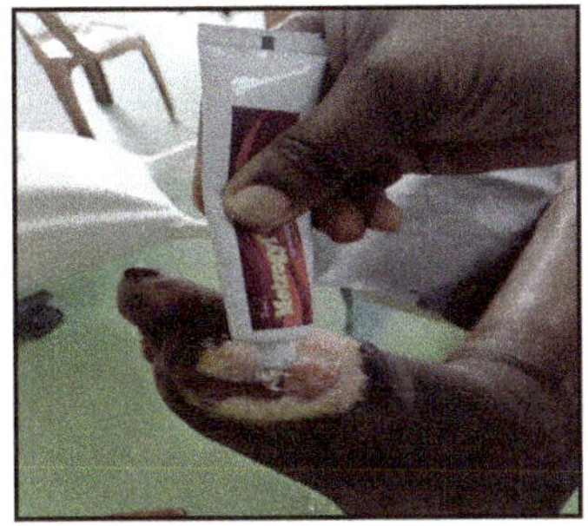 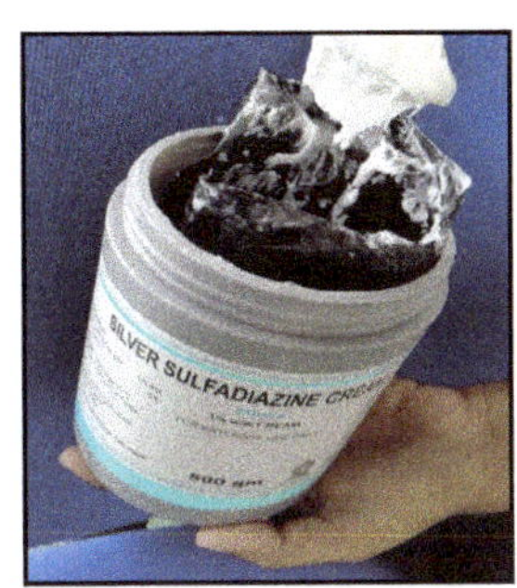

Antiseptic dressings.

Nowadays most antibacterial dressings contain topical antiseptics. Iodine, silver (SSD) and medical grade honey are most popular. It allows wound fluid to drain freely in to the absorbent secondary dressing. Antiseptic dressings are inactive against spores and fungi but effective against wide range of gram positive and negative organisms. Pseudomonas and Proteus shows only a limited sensitivity.

Eg:- Chlorhexidine impregnated tulle dressings (0.5%chlorhexidine acetate) Bactigras – antiseptic parafin impregnated gauze dressings are still used.

Iodine

Iodine is used in two forms. Iodine in cadexomer is released from the starch base (Iodosorb) when it comes in contact with wound exudate.

Iodine in cadexomer has a de-sloughing action. Povidone iodine consists of elemental iodine and synthetic polymer. Iodosorb - cadexomer ointment or powder, 3 g sachet. Powder is cheaper and can be sprinkled on wounds. These must not be used on dry necrotic wounds. Dressing change is done when the colour of powder changes after the release of iodine. Application of Iodosorb daily is not warranted and also uneconomical.

10% betadine solution is only used for surgical scrub and intact skin prep. Alcohol based preparation must not be used on open wound or within the peritoneal cavity. To wash legs, diluted warm water stained with betadine can be used. It is important to wash the legs for at least half an hour in a basin or a bucket. If the patient is bed ridden betadine soaked towels can be applied for half an hour with a rubber mattress underneath.

- Betadine is toxic to fibroblasts, dries the tissues and may cause necrosis and pain.
- It is perhaps best avoided during pregnancy, lactation and in patients with thyroid disorders.

Inodine - Non adherent knitted viscose fabric impregnated with 10% povidone Iodine equivalent to 1% available iodine and polyethylene glycol (provides water soluble environment).

N.B. Iodosorb ; Change the dressing when its colour changes as antiseptic efficacy diminishes.

Silver

Silver is used as a topical antibacterial agent since Roman times. The silver ion (Ag+) is the active antimicrobial agent. Commonly used preparation is Flamazine – Silver Sulphadiazine. Now there are many silver impregnated dressings in the market. Silver should not be used on the face

Effectiveness of silver does not last for more than 7 days. Continuous use of silver containing dressing on chronic wounds should be avoided to prevent local skin discoloration (Face) and development of Argyria. If a net is used it should not remain in place for more than 4 days as granulation tissue may overgrow through causing trauma on removal'

E.g.:- Acticoat - is a silver containing dressing. It consists of absorbent rayon or polyester core sandwiched between two layers of nanocrystalline silver containing polyethylene net. Ideal for partial or full thickness wounds, burns and pressure sores.

Acquacel Ag - This is an absorbent hydro fibre (Sodium carboxy-methyl cellulose which gels on contact with exudate) impregnated with 1.2% ionic silver. Indicated for infected wounds or for wounds with an increased risk of infection.

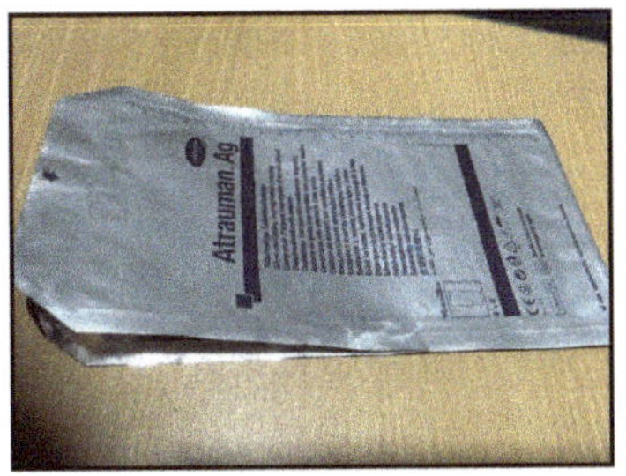
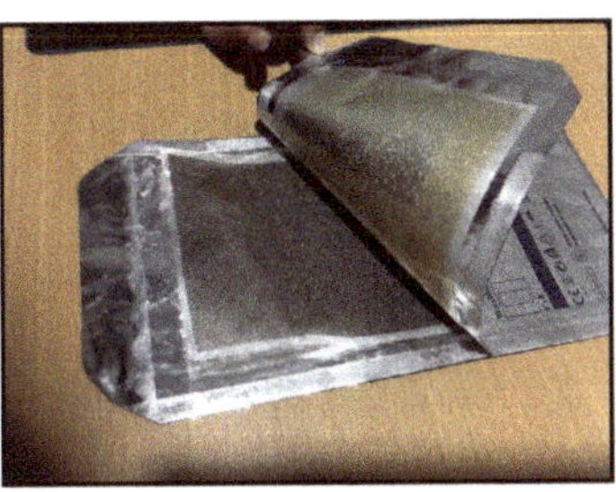

Atrauman Ag - this is a non-adherent polyamide mesh impregnated with neutral triglycerides impregnated with silver.

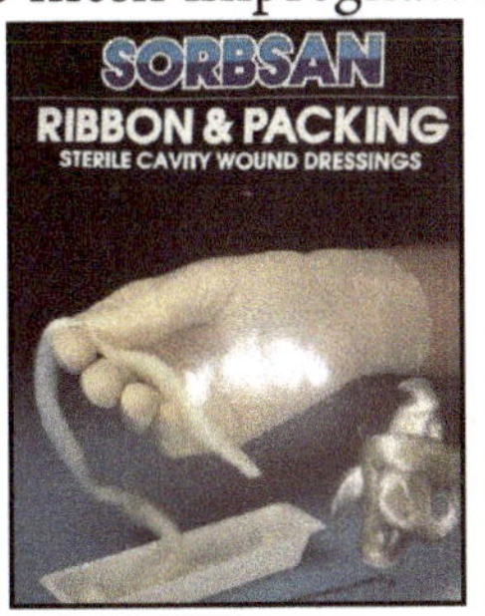

Sorbsan silver packing – calcium alginate cavity packing impregnated with silver for infected and exudating wounds. Silver ions are released on contact with exudate and effectiveness of silver lasts for about7 days.

Polyhexamethylene, guanidine–biocidal (Fungicidal & bactericidal) disinfectant;

PHMB is bactericidal to Escherichia coli. Positively charged PHMB is deadly for the negatively charged cell wall of E.coli.

Chlorhexidine gluconate;

Chlorhexidine 4% solution is used only for the surface skin cleaning but should not use in wound as it is cytotoxic.

Chlorhexidine impregnated tulle 0.5%can be used but they adhere and tissues go through the net after a few days and as it is hydrophobic and water repellent. It causes maceration of peri-wound skin. It is also inactivated by hard water and body fluids and may be cytotoxic to cells.

e.g. Bactigras - Medicated Paraffin gauze containing chlorhexidine acetate 0.5%.

Supportive dressings and bandaging
Compression bandage or hosiery

In persons over the age of 65, 70% of the leg ulcers are due to venous disease. It is important to explain to the patient the etiological factors of venous hypertension which will encourage them to wear support stockings and elevate legs when sedentary. Taking time to explain the aetiology of varicose veins and eventual venous hypertension is important, as the patient will make an attempt to encourage venous return. Aetiology of venous hypertension and varicose veins formation is as follows.

1. Loss of unidirectional blood flow against gravity towards the heart due to incompetence of valves in the long saphenous and short saphenous veins, deep veins, perforators especially at sapheno-femoral junction and sapheno-popliteal junctions.

2. Failure of calf-muscle-foot pump (thigh muscle contractions with in the fascial compartment is also important) which pump blood against the gravity on movement via a system of competent unidirectional valves,

Graduated compression either by bandages or compression hosiery to assist venous return is the mainstay of the conservative treatment in the lower limb venous disease.

Before applying any compression it is important assess blood supply to the limb. If pedal pulses are not present, make sure sharp triphasic or biphasic Doppler ultrasound signals are present. Perhaps ankle brachial pressure index ABPI must be >0.9 before any bandaging done for any requirement.

Folding of stockings in front of the ankle, back of the knee may cause pressure necrosis in the crease or folding lines which may be disastrous in a leg with a compromised circulation. Also rolling of bandages or stockings at thigh or foot ends must be avoided in order to avoid tourniquet effect.

All clinicians, nurse practitioners and wound care specialists must learn to use hand held Doppler probe and learn to assess the quality of sounds and to measure Ankle Brachial Pressure Index. A ratio is calculated between the highest brachial arterial pressure and the highest of ankle pressure measured by Doppler sounds using a BP cuff at the ankle. Blood pressure cuff should not be applied if a large painful ulcer is present at the ankle or deep vein thrombosis is suspected.

Therefore it is important asses the quality of the Doppler sound. The probe is placed at 45 degrees against the arterial flow using ultrasound gel to establish contact with skin over the artery e.g. dorsalis pedis or posterior tibial arteries. Normal sounds are sharp and tri or biphasic. Poor sounds are muffled and monophasic. The triphasic sounds consist of forward systolic, reverse systolic and diastolic flow. ABPI is measured by dividing ankle pressure by the best brachial systolic pressure.

Formation of ulcers in venous hypertension is more common in the gaiter area especially above the medial malleolus where the venous pressure is at its highest.

The common denominator for all sequelae of varicose veins is Venous Hypertension. There are various theories as to how tissue damage and ulceration develops.

1. Pere-capillary fibrin cuff theory. This is formed due to leakage of fibrinogen through dilated capillaries reducing the oxygenation of surrounding tissues as the capillaries are encased with fibrin.
2. Leucocyte entrapment theory. White cell adherence to endothelium releasing inflammatory mediators, cytokines

causing inflammation.

3. Expression of vascular cell adhesion protein 1; VCAM-1, encoded by VCAM 1 gene (vascular cell adhesion molecule) adhesion molecules on the endothelial cells, causing stasis-dermatitis. Also involved is ICAM 1(CD 54) a protein that in humans encoded by ICAM gene.

4. Microangiopathy due to formation of micro emboli in capillaries.

5. Ischemia-reperfusion injury.

6. Pooling of deoxygenated blood in the lower limbs with highest pressure in the gaiter area.

Therefore the use of compression hosiery, elevation of limbs when sedentary is important to aid venous return, to reverse the effects of chronic venous insufficiency such as oedema , reduce exudate and aid healing of ulcers.

Compression bandages or hosiery assist the calf muscles in their pumping action.

Compression bandage can be applied over a primary wound dressing. May need to change these bandages from time to time to maintain proper compression levels and proper shape. These facts when explained to patients, result in good outcomes.

Standard compression levels are as follows. Compression bandages are classified as long stretch (100% extensibility, applied at 50% stretch and exert compression even at rest), short stretch (non elasticated) or multilayer. Most bandages are applied over a layer of orthopaedic wool or soft roll (2 layer system). All bandages should be applied from toes up with leg elevated and all superficial veins empty, just like the way it is done after injecting for sclerosent (STD) compression therapy.

A well-known multilayer system is Chairing cross four layer system [19]. (orthopaedic wool/cotton crepe/elastic extensible/cohesive bandage)

Measurement of ankle circumference is vital for safe compression. Most of the bandage systems are designed to fit ankle circumferences of 18-25 cm. Ankles less the 18cm in circumference needs more wool or soft roll padding to reduce the pressure to safer levels as the pressure exerted by a bandage of a given width increases with the reduction of the circumference (La Place's Law).Bandages should always be applied with the leg elevated with veins emptied and toes up to prevent swelling of the fore foot.

Most clinicians use figure of eight or spiral technique with 50% overlap. It is important to hold the roll of the bandage always outside the bandage to facilitate bandaging and feel the tension of the stretch. Whenever you cut the bandage, slip the blunt rounded knob or fang of the scissors under the fabric against the skin in order to avoid cuts to the skin underneath.

Class 1 -14-17 mm Hg moderate compression for superficial and early varices.
Class 2 - 18-24 mm Hg medium compression for varices of medium severity venous leg ulcers.
Class3 - 25-35 mm Hg high compression for gross varices and post thrombotic syndrome.
It is advisable to teach the patient how to use these devices.

19 John Mears and Christine Moffatt wound care bandaging technique in the treatment of leg ulcers29 Oct.2002 Nursing Times vol 98 issue 44 page 44.

Chapter 12

Advanced wound dressing techniques

VAC therapy- Vacuum Assisted Closure for highly exuding wounds.

VAC therapy or Vacuum Assisted Closure therapy is a method of sealed surface wound suction using suction pump.[20] The topical negative pressure is set at -125mmHg and can be titrated according to the amount of exudate. VAC therapy is used when exudate is so excessive and cannot be handled by any other method of dressing. Wound is packed with open-cell foam dressing, sealed with an adhesive film and foam cells are connected via a tube to a negative pressure pump. Foam dressing is changed every 48 hours.

Advantages are:

- Remove excess fluid.
- Increase oxygenation and nutrient delivery by improving circulation as pressure within the capillaries is higher.
- Remove matrix metalloproteinases which cause breakdown of collagen and other proteins.
- Reduce local wound oedema.
- Anti-microbial activity.

20 S. Thomas, A.M.Andrews, N.P.Hey and S.Bourgoise ; JTV 1999 Vol. 9 No 6 Pages127-132.

n Morykwas M J.et al Vacuum Assisted Closure: state of basic research and physiologic foundation. Plastic Reconstr.Surg. 2006; 117 (suppl.) S 1216.

It is now believed that intermittent suction of repeated cycles (cycles of 5 minute suction on and 2 minutes off) gives better results.

VAC Therapy should not be used in patients on antiplatelet therapy or anticoagulation. The suction foam should not be placed over exposed organs and blood vessels or secreting ducts.   Initial pain can be controlled with reducing the suction pressure.

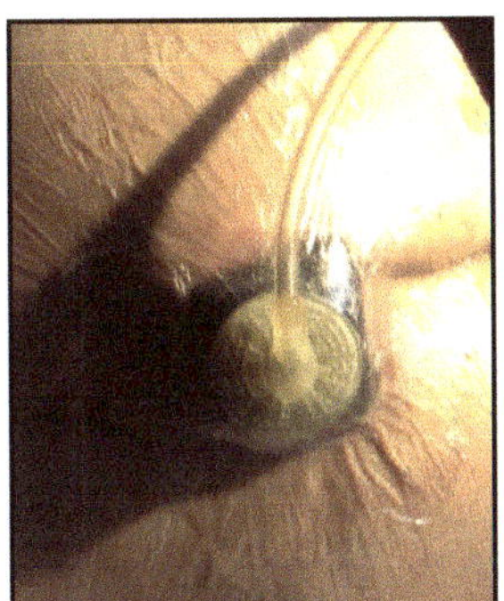 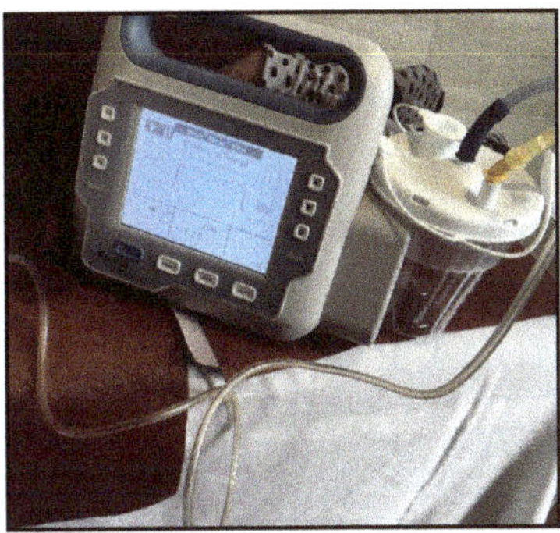

Maggot Therapy;

Medi-flys or maggots are sterile larvae that hatch from eggs laid by laboratory reared flies. Lucilia sericata (green bottles) or Lucilia cuprina are the flies commonly used. Maggots produce powerful proteolytic enzymes that break down slough and necrotic tissues and may ingest bacteria. Maggots has been used for wound debridement since Napoleonic times and among the clinicians they are known as the "world's smallest surgeons". Maggots can be applied as free range larvae or as maggots.

It is important to council the patient as they may reject the treatment out of hand, due to repugnance or due to the so called "Yuk factor". The clinician must explain that they do not multiply or go round the body but uses an enzymatic action and all will be counted and removed in full in 72 hours. Hydrocolloid sheets to form a shallow chamber with hole made to introduce larvae or a net boot can be used. Both systems must be sealed with a hydrocolloid sheet or rim. If hydrocolloid sheet cannot be used the periwound skin can be sealed and protected with strips of a bandage impregnated with zinc paste.

Maggot's therapy should not be used in patients taking anticoagulants or antiplatelets.

They should not be used over large blood vessels, bowels fistulas and sinuses communicating with interior organs or peritoneal cavity.

Larvae secretions kill or prevent growth of Streptococcus Lancefield group A & B, and Staphylococcus aureus. Some activity has been detected against Pseudomonas species and MRSA.

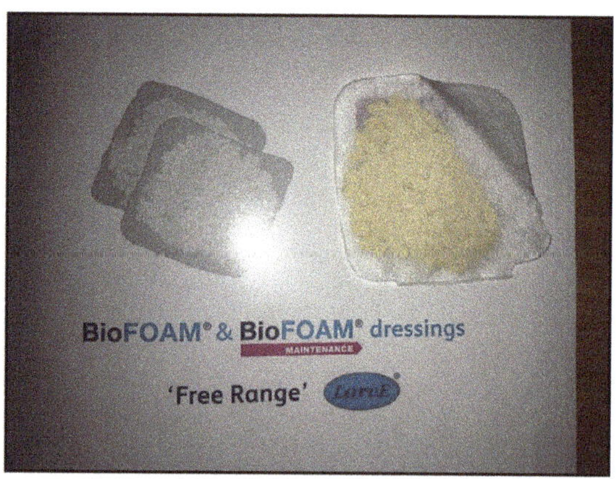

Chapter 13

Wound closure

Skin closure

Simple clean incised operative wound can be closed by primary suturing metal clips, skin bonding glue (fast setting cyanoacrylates) or steri strips (adhesive strips). Application of steri strips must be done accurately. Use a non-toothed forceps. Hold the strip at one end flat at right angles, apply the sticky side down and paste one side of the wound and advance the skin on the opposite side with the gloved fingertip to close the gap before pasting the other end of the strip to the opposite skin.

Various suturing methods are available.

Interrupted
    I.Simple sutures.
    II. Mattress sutures (vertical or parallel).

Sutures used are non-absorbable monofilament synthetic polymers e.g. polypropylene (proline) and nylon (Ethilon). They are least like to lead to infection (c.f - Braided sutures). Sutures should be not too tight as crosshatching may leave an unsightly scar. All non-absorbable sutures on skin must be removed when the wound is healed.

Continuous suture

I.   Long wounds. A continuous through loop suture can be used in long class one or two wounds.

II.   Subcuticular suture with an absorbable material has a better cosmetic outcome and is widely used in paediatric practices.

It is difficult to remove sutures due to lack of cooperation by the child. Suture material used here should be absorbable polyglactin 910 (Vicryl Rapide).

It is not advisable to use a continuous suture in class three or four wounds as abscess formation is possible. They need interrupted sutures. If any collection occurs blood, pus or serum it can be by drained just by removing a couple of sutures and probing the wound. A seroma can be easily aspirated with a needle and a syringe.

Traumatic Wounds

All traumatic wounds must be irrigated cleaned and if necessary drained before closing. It is always important to think about tetanus and antibiotic cover. Mud contaminated friction wounds and wounds with foreign bodies and devitalised tissues will need proper debridement under anaesthesia.

Skin grafting

I. Pinch grafting; good for smaller wounds in the leg or foot where cosmetic aspect is not important. A local anaesthetic, a syringe and number 23 blade is all that is required. Skin can be tented with the needle tip under local anaesthesia and a small slice of skin taken. Middle of the skin is almost full thickness and periphery is partial thickness. These are placed in the wound. Even if all pinches do not take the rest will epithelialize from the edges to cover the wound.

II. Split skin grafting; Donor area usually is antero-lateral aspect of the thigh. The graft consists of split skin and a variable amount of dermis and taken using the Humby hand held skin graft knife or powered dermatome.

The optimum harvest is 0.35 mm thick. The use of a number 10 (0.37mm thick) or 15 (0.39mm thick) scalpel blade as a "feeler gauge" to measure the appropriate setting for the hand held knife is reasonably accurate. Adjust the knife to a setting just wide enough to permit the scalpel blade. Lubricate and tense the donor skin with skin graft boards before skin graft knife is applied.

Exposed bone or tendon without paratenon is not suitable for skin grafting. For large recipient areas the graft should be meshed using a blade or mesher which comes with the powered dermatome. Meshing also prevent graft lifting off the wound bed by underlying haematoma.

Flaps- Larger musculo-fascial defect can be covered using pedicled flaps based on perforating blood vessel at its base or free flaps harvested from elsewhere in the body using microvascular techniques.

Post-operative dressings;

Most commonly applied dressings are simple, low adherent waterproof thin dressings. Island dressings with adhesive borders are also popular. It is important that the adhesive border is not under any drag or tension as blistering may occur. Others are thin hydrocolloid sheets such as Duoderm, impregnated film island dressings such as Tegaderm with betadine. Vapour permeable adhesive film dressing with absorbent pad (Opsite Post op) or absorbent perforated dressing with adhesive border (Premi-Pore) can be used post operatively for slightly oozing wounds.

When suturing facial wounds, monofilament fine, non-absorbable suture should be used without any tension with regular gaps for steri-strips. In order to avoid unsightly cross hatching marks, sutures should be removed in 3 days, leaving original steristrips and replacing sutures by further steristrips.

Needles used for skin or subcutaneous suturing are cutting (c.f. round bodied with tapering needle in bowel surgery). Forceps used are toothed as non-toothed forceps cause pressure necrosis. In any case, skin and tissues should be handled without tooth marks or any trauma. "Hook and lever", "eversion and counter pressure" methods are used with tips of forceps kept open at most times. There should be no tension in tying knots as pressure necrosis may cause unsightly cross hatching marks.

Use the finest suture that will hold the wound together. Absorbable polyglactin (vicryl) suture should be used to approximate subcutaneous fat or fascia (e.g. scarpa) to avoid a dead space, a potential space for a haematoma or seroma.

Needle tip must entter the skin at right angles to avoid superficial slicing sideways. Skin edges must not gape or overlap.

Modern sutures are atraumatic i.e. needle is swaged on to the suture. With monofilament suture material it is best to use a double throw at the first knot followed by 5 single throws. All throws should be square reef knots to avoid slip knots. At the end of suturing it is important to roll a gauze roll over length of the wound to squeeze out any blood left in the wound before applying the wound dressing.

There has to be a good reason for the first dressing to be changed or disturbed. If the dressing strike through with exudate or blood, or local or systemic signs of infection is present in the wound, then the wound should be inspected.

Removal of sutures

Most medical students are asked "when is the best time to removes sutures from a wound?" The best answer is "When the wound is healed". Healing of wound depends on the site and condition of the wound.

Times of healing in different sites in the body. Sutures are removed when the wound is healed.

Site	Approx. No of days
Face	3 days steristrip in-between can be left for a few days more..
Scalp	7 days
Upper limb	7 days
Body above umbilicus	7 days
Below umbilicus	10 to 12 days.
Lower limb	12 to14 days.

If the wound is wet and gaping in between sutures on touch it is better to wait a couple more days

The main principle of removing suture is not to drag exposed infected suture segment through the clean suture tract under the skin. In order to achieve this, one must cut the suture at one end flush with the skin.

Before removing the sutures touch the wound edge gently with finger tips on either side of the incision. If the wound is moist or there is clear gaping between sutures, it should be cleaned with betadine and a new dressing should be applied for 4 more days. If the wound gapes soon after removal of sutures, steristrips can be applied for a further period. Sometimes re-suturing may be necessary under local anaesthesia.

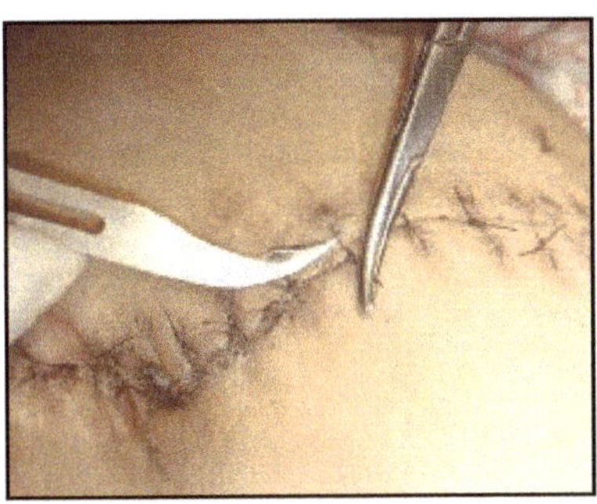

Chapter 14

New biological methods available for promoting wound healing.

These methods are only used for non-healing chronic wounds which are stuck in various stages of wound healing, mostly in the inflammatory phase.

Some products such as growth factors target a specific phase of healing.

Products targeting inflammatory phase. E.g. Promogran inactivate harmful proteases and protect growth factors. Any infection and slough must be cleared for the treatment to be effective.

Products targeting proliferative phase. E.g. Fibroblast attracting platelet derived growth factor (PDGF) and transforming growth factor beta (TGFB).

Becaplermin (Regranex gel), fibroblast growth factor (FGF) promotes fibroblast proliferation and Vascular Endothelial Growth Factor promotes angiogenesis.

Products targeting epithelialisation and remodelling. E.g. epidermal growth factor stimulates **epithelialisation.** Keratinocyte Growth Factor (KGF) induces **proliferation and migration of keratinocytes.** Topical human recombinant Granulocyte Macrophage colony stimulating factor (GM-CSF) promotes **epidermal cell proliferation** and is effective in healing venous leg ulcers.

TGF-b3 (Transforming Growth Factor beta 3 encoded by TGFB3gene) which reduces deposition of collagen may be effective in preventing hypertrophic scars.

Biological products can be classified as follows;

1. Artificial skin substitutes - Alloderm-human cadaver skin.

2. Composite epidermal substitutes – allogenic keratinocytes, fibroblasts-epidermal equivalent).

3. Growth factors - Promogran, Dermograft, and Cell spray.

4. Sterile medicated collagen particles - BioFil-AB particles with antibiotics such as mupirocin and metronidazole,

5. Pharmocol – chemically modified collagen sheets cross linked with glutaraldehyde. These can be used to fill defects in muscular-fascial structures such as adnominal wall. Best to use the sheets without any tension and additional techniques such as component separation by incising and releasing facial sheaths more laterally. There is peculiar smell of this product does not always indicate infection.

6. Strattice Reconstructive Tissue Matrix – This is a non-cross linked porcine-derived acellular (all the cellular material removed) dermal matrix – a biologic mesh (PADM). The resulting mesh like substance provides a scaffolding that supports the growth of healthy new tissue to replace various facial defects.

Not many randomized controlled trials are available for biological products and only a few trials are available for growth factor treatment especially in relation to dose and duration.

Chapter 15

Selection of wound dressings for chronic ulcers

During the healing phases wound will exhibit different tissue types. It is generally accepted there are five main tissue types but as the phases of wound healing overlap, more than one type of tissue may exist in the same wound. No dressing should be used on individuals who are sensitive to or who have had an allergic reaction to the dressing or its components.

Withanage "SINGLE classification" ; Easy to remember classification for medical students.

1. Sloughy wounds.

2. Infected wounds.

3. Necrotic wounds.

4. Granulating wounds.

5. Lumpy granulating wounds. (Proud flesh)

6. Epithelializing wounds.

(S) Sloughy wounds.

These wounds are characterized by the presence of soft necrotic tissue and dead phagocytes. It is yellow in colour. No epithelialisation will take place until slough is completely removed. It is best to irrigate the wound thoroughly with warm saline to identify the correct tissue type. Must differentiate pus produced by an infection from remnants of previously applied wound care products in the wound.

The aim of treatment is de-sloughing and removing excess exudate from the wound.

Hydrocolloid containing gel formers can be used since they hydrate, soften and autolyse necrotic tissue and slough.

Sloughy wounds – superficial, small and dry

Hydrocolloid sheet E.g.: grnuflex, comfeel, duoderm.

Sodium carboxy-methylcellulose (CMC), gelatin, pectin, elastomers and adhesives bonded to a carrier of a semipermeable film or foam sheet to produce a flat adhesive dressing. The dressing forms a gel on contact with wound exudate.

Granuflex; Adhesive hydrocolloid dressing consisting of an inner layer of hydrocolloid within an adhesive polymer matrix and an outer layer of polyurethane foam. It has carboxy-methyl cellulose, pectin and gelatin which gel in contact with exudate by absorbing water.

The adhesive layer forms adhesive gel on contact with exudate. This gel is not mobile or free running and the dressing is waterproof so that the patient can have shower. They can be lightly pressed in to position (e.g. pressure necrosis on the back of the heel) with a minimum overlap of 2 cm onto the normal periwound skin. The sheet can be lifted at a corner to examine the wound as the dressing change will depend on the state of the wound. It is accepted by most clinicians that the dressing should not be left for more than 7 days.

Comfeel plus; this is an absorbent hydrocolloid dressing with a vapour permeable film backing and an adhesive boarder. It can be shaped for use on uneven areas such as elbows and knees.

Duoderm; It is a thinner hydrocolloid sheet. The adhesive layer contains elastomeric properties which has the ability to contain wound exudate.

Use Hydrocolloid gel, paste or fibre with a secondary dressing for deeper wounds and Hydrocolloid sheet for more superficial wounds.

Fibre is useful for cavities, sinuses or undermining wounds.

Sloughy wounds small and moist; most need a secondary dressing;

Hydrocolloid paste is also now available e.g. GranuGel paste as a good debriding agent.

Hydrocolloid sheet – Granuflex also can be used.

Hydro fibre –e.g. Aquacel – soft sterile non-woven pad composed of Hydrofibre (Sodium carboxymethylcellulose-CMC).

Hydrogels. E.g. Aciform cool, ionic (NA) hydrogel sheet donate or absorb fluid depending on the moisture available in the wound.

Manuka honey; e.g. Activon. Medical grade honey can also be used for autolytic debridement. Honey can be used even when the wound is infected.

Deep cavity wet wounds with yellow brown slough.

Hydrogels; e.g. Sherisorb, Intrasite gel. It is a transparent aqueous (partially hydrated) gel containing 2.3% modified Carboxy methylcellulose polymer with propylene glycol 20%, as a humectant (retain or preserve moisture) and a preservative.

Hydrogel donate water to dry wounds and also absorbs excess exudate (give & take).

Sloughy - Highly exuding wounds;

Alginates; A brown seaweed phaeophyceae can be used for highly exuding wounds. It contain 100% Calcium alginate 80:20, Ca: Na alginate which dissolves in contact with wound to form a hydrophilic gel.

Mannuronic acid rich Kaltostat gel is washable and Guluronic rich Sorbsan gel is pickable rather than washable. Alginates absorbs 15 to 20 times their weight of fluid. Due to the presence of calcium, alginates has haemostatic properties. Therefore they can be used in incision drainage fresh wounds such as perianal, pilonidal and ischiorectal abscesses following incision and drainage.

More extensive slough in the wound larva (maggot) therapy should be considered.

Extensive slough with unmanageable exudation using above mentioned techniques can be treated with topical negative pressure. This is a sealed surface wound suction technique also known as vacuum assisted closure (VAC therapy). These improve circulation due to relatively positive capillary pressure. Sub-atmospheric pressure removes excessive exudate, bacteria, metalloproteinases (which break collagen and proteins).

(I) Infected wounds

The main aim is to reduce bacterial load. These are usually wet with excessive exudate. Cultures for sensitivity should be carried out but systemic or local antibiotics are not given unless there are generalized clinical symptoms and spreading signs such as cellulites, lymphangitis, lymphadenitis and pyrexia. Most of the dressings used will require a secondary dressing.

Infected wounds - Shallow and wet.

i. Cadexomer Iodine ointment or dressing with Iodosorb powder.

Iodosorb; Iodine containing yellow brown microspheres (Iodosorb) in sachets; 0.1-0.3 mm in diameter formed from a three dimensional network of cadexomer – a chemically modified starch. The hydrophilic beads contain 0.9% w/w of iodine which is held firmly within the structure of the polymer and are not liberated in the dry state.

Iodine is released when beads take up water. By capillary action bacteria and slough become trapped between the beads e.g. Iodosorb. Dressing lose colour when saturated with exudate. That is the time to redress the wound.

i. Metronidazole containing colourless transparent aqueous gel ; each gram contains 10mg of metronidazole in a base of betadex, edetate disodium, hydroxymethyl cellulose, methyl paraben, niacinamide, phenoxyethanol, propylene glycol, propyl paraben and purified water.

ii. Iodosorb plus metrogel

iii. Atrauman Ag. Non adherent polyamide mesh wound contact layer with 1 mm pores and impregnated with neutral triglycerides coated with metallic silver. Dressings can be left for 4 days. Excellent as a "touch and kill dressing for contaminated, colonised and infected wounds.

iv. Chlorhexidine tulle e.g. Bactigras. No tulle should be left in the wound for more than 3 days as granulation tissue grow through and will cause trauma on removal.

All need a secondary dressing.

Infected wounds; Deep and wet.

1. Iodosorb with metrogel (beads will lose its colour when saturated with exudate – change the dressing)

2. Aquacel Ag ; absorbent white fibrous dressing composed of Hydrofibre (sodium CMC) impregnated with 1.2% Ionic Silver. Aquacell Ag forms a coherent soft gel on contact with exudate.

Both need a secondary dressing (A pad or a retention dressing)

If there is excessive exudate VAC Negative pressure therapy should be considered.

(N) Necrotic wounds

Presence of dead or de-vitalized tissue, black or brown discoloration. The wound cannot heal until all necrotic tissue is removed. There is only a subtle difference in the dressing used for Sloughy and necrotic wounds. The dressing must create a moist environment, hydrate, soften and autolyse necrotic tissue.

Small superficial and dry necrotic wound

For black necrotic patches adhesive hydrocolloid sheets are the best. It is an occlusive dressing which offer an effective barrier to microorganisms. Outer layer is made of polyurethane foam. E.g. Granuflex.

Extensive, deep necrotic wound with moderate exudate.

1. A large hydrocolloid sheet e.g. Granuflex.(But without side cavitation).

2. Amorphous Hydrogel with a secondary dressing e.g. Intrasite gel. Sherisorb.

3. Actiform cool; ionic non adherent hydrogel sheet, donate moisture or absorb exudate.

4. Manuka Honey (Activon) Antibacterial medical grade. (C.I. bee venom allergy). Monitor blood sugar levels in diabetics. Available as tulle dressings as well.

Secondary Dressings

Selection of secondary dressings for primary wound dressings of necrotic or sloughy wounds.

1. If the wound is dry; an occlusive dressing to reduce water and vapour loss. E.g. Opsite, Flexigrid.
2. Lightly exuding wound; a perforated film absorbent dressing. E.g. Melolin, Telfa.
3. If there is significant exudate; an absorbent pad can be used, e.g. Allevyn, Lyoform polyurethane pads.

(G) Granulating wound.

Chronic - low to medium exudate.

Alginate sheet e.g. Sorbsan
Hydrocolloid sheet e.g. Granuflex extra thin.
Polyurethane foam dressing. E.g. Lyofoam.
Extra absorbency Hydrocolloid sheet. (E.g.Granuflex E)
Chronic wound with granulations - medium to high exudate;

Alginate sheet, rope or ribbon (e.g. sorbsan)
Polyurethane foam dressing. e.g. Lyoform.
Surgical tissue loss. E.g. pilonidal sinus infection, excised as block and laid open. Granulating cavity foam dressing. Silastic foam.

Silastic foam is supplied as monomer 500g and catalyst 40 ml. They are mixed in the ratio of 10 ml monomer to 0.6 ml catalyst. The mixture is stirred and poured into the cavity. Soft pliable slightly absorbent white foam block is formed to fit into the cavity without any internal pressure. This block can be washed and reused but it is better to redo the packing when the volume of the wound is reduced due to contraction.

As a general rule no cavity should be tightly packed with any dressing as it prevents wound or cavity contraction.

(L) Lumpy granulation wound. "Proud Flesh"

This is also known as exuberant granulation tissue formation and is the excessive growth of granulation tissue which grows above the skin level. Hyper granulation usually occurs due to prolong stimulation and angiogenesis. Healing process is arrested as it will make it impossible for epithelialisation. Excessive irritation, infection, inflammation and hypoxia are some of the causes responsible for proud flesh.

Silver nitrate sticks coagulate tissue and kills bacteria. Tissue collapses almost immediately but may set up further inflammation and exudation.　It is important to repeat the treatment a few times at different sittings.

Sharp debridement with excision of granulation tissue to the level of skin and applying an occlusive pressure dressing may work.

Surgical lasers; can also be applied. These remove granulation tissue and cauterize small blood vessels.

Sharp debridement is possibly the best, but it recurs. Excision and cauterization of the base with silver nitrate sticks gives good results. Wash the tissues with warm water following cautery.

(E) Epithelializing wounds

Epithelializing - Clean wounds with low exudate.

1. Semipermeable film e.g. Opsite.
2. Hydrocolloid sheet e.g. Granuflex.

Epithelializing - Clean wounds with medium to high exudate;

1. Alginate sheet e.g. Sorbsan.
2. Extr-absorbancy hydrocolloid sheet. Granuflex E.
3. Hydrophilic polyurethane foam.

Chapter 16

Universal precautions in wound care

Normally skin as a part of the innate immune system, is the first defensive barrier or primary line of defence. It not only prevents the pathogens from entering the body but also create an inhospitable environment for pathogens to grow.

It is important to note that in a wound, the first barrier of defence is not the skin which has already been breached but the inflammatory reaction known as acute inflammation created by the innate immune system.

Eventually with the invasion of bacterial antigens, adaptive immune response i.e. antibody mediated humoral immunity and cell mediated immunity will take over.

During adaptive immune response, cells involved are T lymphocytes and B lymphocytes. There are two types of T cells. T killer (cytotoxic) cells and T helper cells which helps to activate B Lymphocytes and macrophages (from Monocytes). B Lymphocytes produce daughter cells which mature into plasma cells which in turn produce 5 classes of antibodies (IgM, IgG, IgA, IgD, IgE).

Pre-operative skin preparation.

Hair clipping should be carried out just before surgery. Shaving itself causes skin abrasions and has been largely abandoned in the West. If shaver is used it should be carried out as close to surgery as possible.

In painful conditions like perianal, ischio-rectal or pilonidal abscesses, it is best to prepare the operation site under anaesthesia, general or spinal.

Operation site skin is routinely cleansed before surgery in order to reduce the microorganisms present on the skin and reduce surgical site infections. Minimum of 4 inch overlap should be allowed for accidental displacement of drapes. Edge of drapes must be accurately placed on the prepared area without dragging across the unprepared skin. Commonly used antiseptics are Povidone iodine and chlorohexidine. Some surgeons use Betadine impregnated soaks for one minute after cutting through the skin.

a   0.1% Povidone Iodine in 70% alcohol.

b.   0.5% chlorohexidine in 70% alcohol (methylated sprit) is possibly superior to Povidone Iodine[20].

Waste Disposal

It is important to discard infective materials and dressings into designated clinical waste disposal units. "Hampshire dressing technique" is a useful method in collecting infective materials. Here a plastic bag is used as a glove to remove the soil dressings. The dressings are held through the bottom of the bag and the bag is turned inside out over the dressings and discarded.

This method is now commonly used in food industry especially in roadside restaurants in most developing countries as a non-touch technique at the outlets. Before using this method you have to make sure the clinician has disposed sharps – needles and scalpels to the sharps bin. If not the nurse must go through the material with a tissue forceps and discard such material appropriately.

20 Dumville J C, McFalane.E, Edwards.P. Lipp.A, Liu.Z Preoperative skin anticeptics preventing surgical wound infections after clean surgery.Cochrane database of system reviews 2015 Issue 4, Art No. CD 00340, pub 4 Cochrane library.

Perhaps it is best for doctors to discard needles and blades by themselves into appropriate boxes after they finish with suturing or wound debridement.

Asepsis is of paramount importance in all wound dressings. Staff should not transfer infections to the wound or from one patient to another by strictly following standard aseptic technique. In developing countries due to economic reasons ordinary unsterile disposable gloves are used to do the dressings which only protect the staff and possibly cross infection but not the patient. In these situations Steri gel application on the outside of the glove maybe useful. It has been observed that untrained nurses touch door handles, curtains etc. during the procedure, perhaps due to shortage of staff and poor training.

The staff must use Standard Precautions. E.g. gloves, goggles and gowns as needed. (The three Gs'). The staff also must not walk across the ward with dressings in hand looking for the appropriate bin placed at the end of the ward. Hence the importance of a well prepared wound trolley. No one should be allowed to walk between two sterile areas. It is also important to request the patient not touch the clean areas.

Patient's dignity and privacy must be maintained at all times by drawing the curtains adequately around the patient and a "runner" nurse should be present. They must have a small trolley prepared with disposable bags and boxes for bedside dressings or use the designated "procedure room" in the ward. For larger wounds, a septic theatre (a mini OT) can be used.

A syringe can be used for irrigation of wounds with either warm water or warmed sterile saline. Cold water should be avoided if at all possible. Moistened gauze held in forceps can be used to wipe out slough and moist exudates. Insensitive dead tissue within the wound can be removed by sharp dissection remaining within the necrotic area without encroaching on the sensitive wound edge or inject a local anaesthetic to lift the necrotic eschar. All staff must watch patient's facial expression to make sure this process is carried out without any distress or pain to the patient.

If the process is painfull or wounds are extensive close to vital structures perhaps it is best preparethe patient for general or spinal anaesthesia.

It is important to recognise the newly formed rim of pink epithelial tissue at the edges of the wound to prevent any damage to this delicate, newly formed neo-epithelium.

Chapter 17

Economic Usage Of Dressings And Affordability

The National Health Service of developing countries do not provide expensive dressings. As a result, patients are regularly asked to purchase their own. Clinicians must think about the cost of dressings, affordability and wastage caused by inappropriate use. For example, for a wound which needs to be dressed daily, it is not worth using a Hydrocolloid Sheet (Rs.1200). When patients require fresh dressings daily, the use of Metrogyl with a secondary dressing has become a popular alternative.

Additionally, before prescribing dressings, clinicians must assess both the affordability of patients and the funds available to the unit.

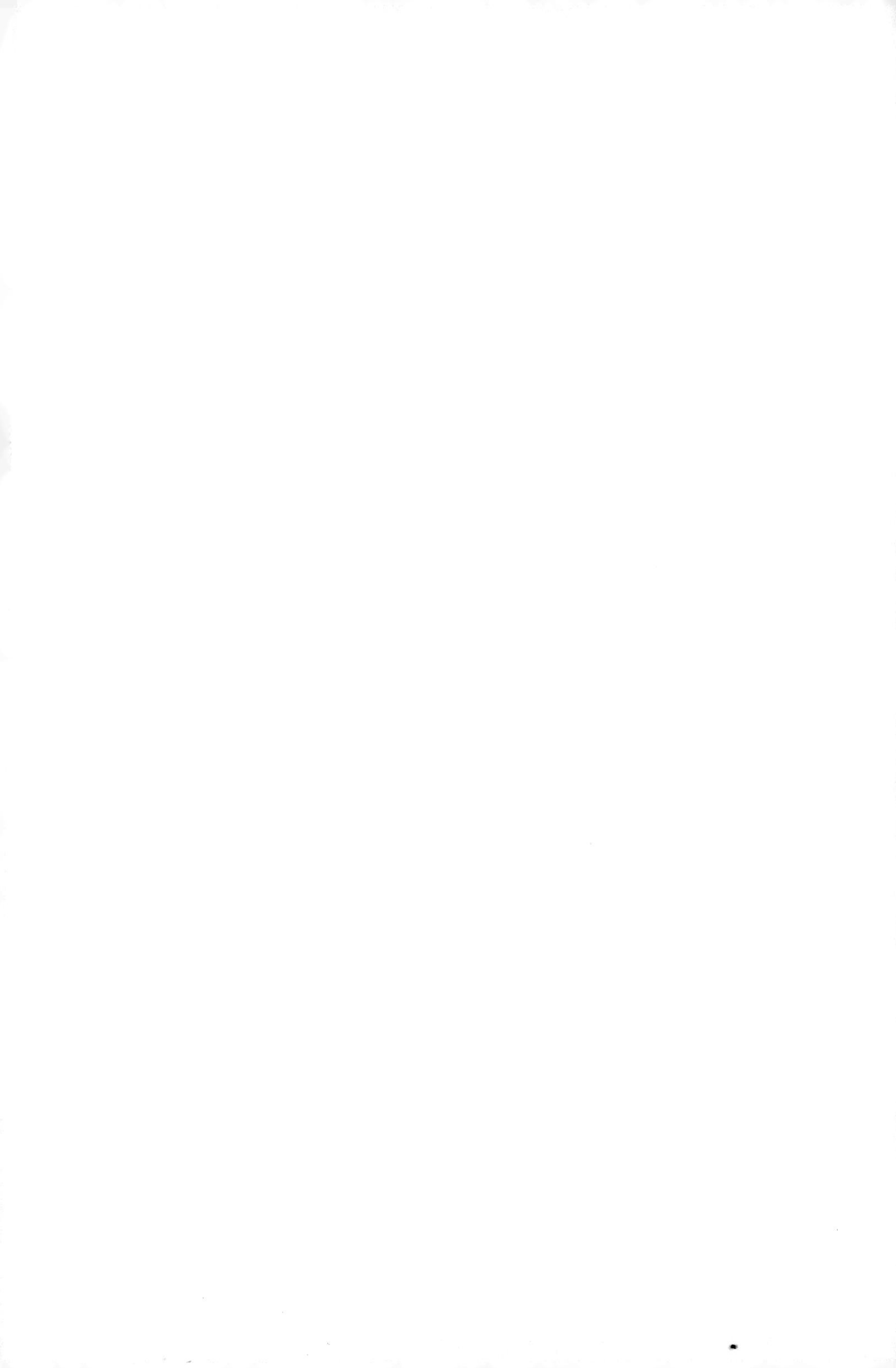